Table of Contents

INTRODUCTION

CHAPTER 1: AN INTRO TO THE LOW-FODMAP DIET

WHAT ARE FODMAPS?
WHAT HAPPENS WHEN WE EAT FODMAPS?

CHAPTER 2: BENEFITS OF THE LOW-FODMAP DIET

WHO SHOULD FOLLOW THE LOW-FODMAP DIET?
WHAT IS IBS?
HOW DOES THE LOW-FODMAP DIET WORK?
BENEFITS OF THE LOW-FODMAP DIET

CHAPTER 3: GETTING STARTED

BEFORE YOU START
FOLLOWING THE DIET AND MAINTAINING YOUR NUTRITION
THINGS TO AVOID
EXAMPLE SHOPPING LIST

CHAPTER 4: BREAKFAST RECIPES

STRAWBERRY CHIA PUDDING
BREAKFAST SMOOTHIE
SPINACH AND SALMON OMELETTE
VEGETABLE OMELET OR SCRAMBLE
CHOCOLATE PORRIDGE
BREAKFAST WRAP
BANANA PANCAKES

Green Smoothie
French Toast with Banana and Pecans
Tofu Breakfast Scramble

CHAPTER 5: LUNCH AND DINNER RECIPES

Rice-Based Recipes:
Salmon Fried Rice
Japanese Rice/Sushi Balls
Pasta-Based Recipes:
Baked Chicken Alfredo Pasta
Spaghetti Bolognese
Soups and Stews:
Lamb Stew:
Salads:
Moroccan-Inspired Chicken Salad with an Orange Dressing
Other Recipes:
Mini Savory Crepes
Lamb Kebabs
Chicken Enchiladas

CHAPTER 6: TASTY SNACK RECIPES

Lemon Zucchini Muffins:
Garlic Bread
Frozen Yogurt Bark
Chicken Quinoa Meatballs
Lemon Coconut Cupcakes
Salted Caramel Pumpkin Seeds
Falafels

CHAPTER 7: MEATLESS MEALS

Vegetarian Recipes:
Unique Vegetable Pizza

Pumpkin Carrot Risotto
Fennel Carrot Soup
Vegan Recipes:
Lentil and Rice Bowl
Kale and Olive Pasta
Chinese Noodle Soup
Indian Spinach Tofu Curry
Spinach Eggplant Pasta

CHAPTER 8: WHY IS THIS DIET NOT WORKING FOR ME?

CONCLUSION

© Copyright 2019 by Lisa McGill - All rights reserved.

This eBook is provided with the sole purpose of providing relevant information on a specific topic for which every reasonable effort has been made to ensure that it is both accurate and reasonable. Nevertheless, by purchasing this eBook you consent to the fact that the author, as well as the publisher, are in no way experts on the topics contained herein, regardless of any claims as such that may be made within. As such, any suggestions or recommendations that are made so purely for entertainment value. It is recommended that you always consult a professional before undertaking any of the advice or techniques discussed within.

This is a legally binding declaration that is considered both valid and fair by both the Committee of Publishers Association and the American Bar Association and should be considered as legally binding within the United States.

The reproduction, transmission, and duplication of any of the content found herein, including any specific or extended information will be done as an illegal act regardless of the end form the information ultimately takes. This includes copied versions of the work both physical, digital, and audio unless express consent of the Publisher is provided beforehand. Any additional rights reserved.

Furthermore, the information that can be found within the pages described forthwith shall be considered both accurate and truthful when it comes to the recounting of facts. As such, any use, correct or incorrect, of the provided information will render the Publisher free of responsibility as to the actions taken outside of their direct purview. Regardless, there are zero scenarios where the original author or the Publisher can be deemed liable in any fashion for any damages or hardships that may result from any of the information discussed herein.

Additionally, the information in the following pages is intended only for informational purposes and should thus be thought of as universal. As befitting its nature, it is presented without assurance regarding its prolonged validity or interim quality. Trademarks that are mentioned are done without written consent and can in no way be considered an endorsement from the trademark holder.

Introduction

Congratulations on downloading *The Low-FODMAP Diet*, and thank you for doing so!

The following chapters will discuss the basics of the diet, its health benefits, and easy recipes that will help you adopt this diet into your lifestyle.

The low-FODMAP diet is the most common diet used by people who suffer from IBS, as it helps alleviate their symptoms. Although the exact cause of IBS is not yet known, this book delves into how and why high-FODMAP foods can contribute to the discomfort and unfavorable symptoms IBS sufferers experience. The first few chapters will also discuss ways to maximize your results with this diet, what you should expect as you move forward, and things to avoid while on the diet.

The majority of the book holds a variety of recipes that will help you get started on this diet and will make the transition from your current diet to the low-FODMAP diet a little easier. I have listed quite a few main meal recipes for meat-lovers, as well as people who are vegetarian or vegan. Each recipe has been reviewed by a dietician and comes with the cooking method and a detailed list of ingredients you will use. The recipes also come with suggested serving size. Sticking to the proper serving sizes of raw ingredients when making a low-FODMAP meal will help your gut feel healthy much faster! Each recipe also comes with low-FODMAP shopping tips that will help you find the right ingredients and ensure that they are suitable for your new gut diet! These tips will also include ways to make your meals vegan or gluten-free if that is what you desire. The alternatives will help you adapt the meals in this book to your lifestyle and diet.

Thanks again for choosing this book, and good luck! Every effort was made to ensure it is full of as much useful information as possible. Please enjoy!

Chapter 1: An Intro to the Low-FODMAP Diet

What Are FODMAPs?

FODMAPs are a set of short-chain carbohydrates that are more difficult to digest than other carbohydrates we ingest. The acronym FODMAP stands for Fermentable Oligo-, Di-, Mono-saccharides, and Polyols. Common FODMAPs in a regular diet include:
- Galatians: large amounts of this are found in legumes.
- Fructose: a simple carb; found in many vegetables and fruits and helps build most added sugar molecules
- Polyols: Sugar alcohols like xylitol, sorbitol, maltitol, and mannitol. They are found in some fruits and vegetables and are often used as sweeteners.
- Lactose: A carb that is commonly found in dairy items like milk.
- Fructans: Found in many foods, including grains like wheat, spelled, rye and barley.

FODMAPs can be found in a wide variety of foods but some foods are more well-known for being high-FODMAP. The following foods are examples of high-FODMAP foods:

- Contain Lactose: regular and low-fat milk and yogurt; soft cheeses like ricotta, cream cheese, and cottage cheese; ice cream, and custard.

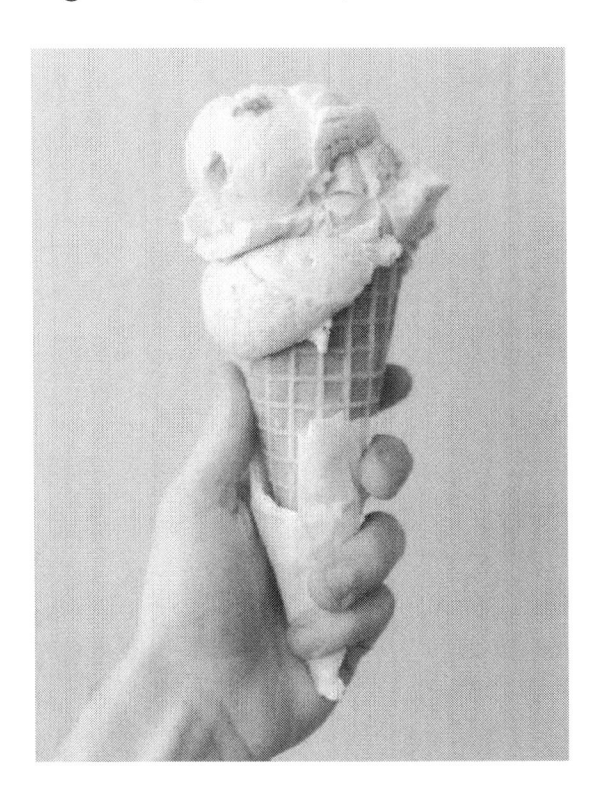

- High in Fructose: fruits like mangoes, pears, cherries, apples, watermelon, or canned fruits marinated in fruit juices; vegetables like sugar snap peas, asparagus, and artichokes; sweeteners like honey and high-fructose corn syrup.
- Contain Fructans and Galacto-oligosaccharides: grains like wheat, rye, and their products; fruits like watermelon, peaches, and persimmons; vegetables like onions, garlic, artichokes, and legumes (baked beans, kidney beans, etc.); and

other products such as inulin—a form of supplemental fiber.

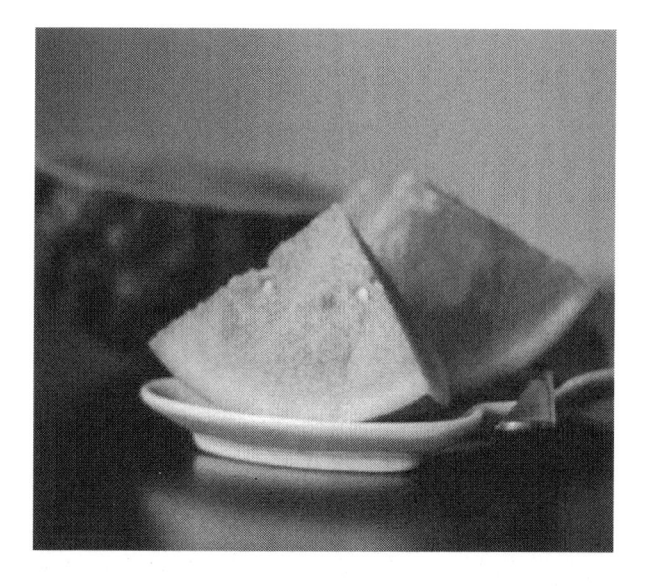

- Contain Sorbitol (Polyol): fruits like apples, blackberries, nectarines, pears, apricots, and plums; beverages like apple juice and pear juice.
- Contain Mannitol (Polyol): vegetables like cauliflower, sugar snap peas, and mushrooms; fruits like watermelon.
- Contain both Sorbitol and Mannitol (Polyols): sweet candies like sugar-free gum, some hard candies, and some chocolate.

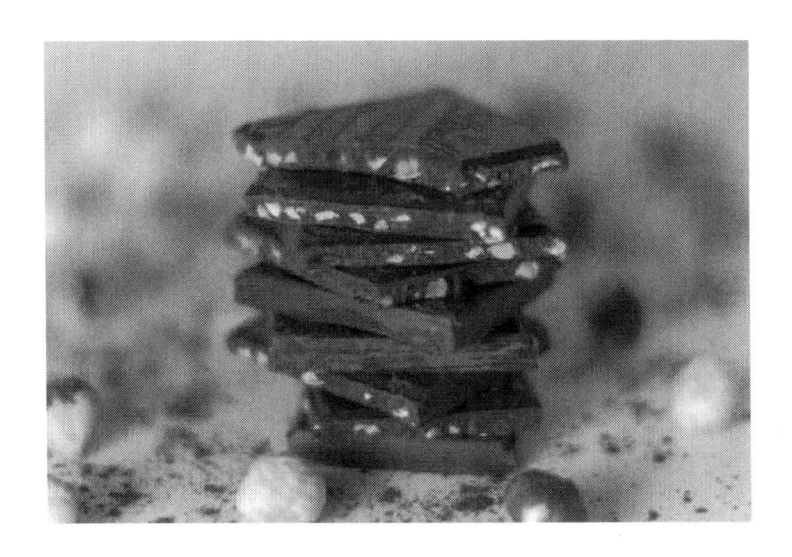

What Happens When We Eat FODMAPs?

Since FODMAP molecules are so resistant to digestion, they are not easily absorbed into the bloodstream. They can travel unchanged throughout the entire length of the intestine and can encourage different parts of your digestive system to draw more water than necessary from your bloodstream. This can result in runny and watery bowel movements in individuals whose systems are sensitive to FODMAPs.

As mentioned above, FODMAP molecules can travel to the end of the digestive tract where most good and helpful gut bacteria, or microflora, reside. There, the bacteria are unsure of what to do with the high amounts of undigested carbs, so they use the molecules as fuel. This respiration process (the biological process of producing energy from organic substances) results in the production of excess byproducts, like hydrogen gas, that can cause more indigestion symptoms.

Since FODMAPs themselves are not harmful (only people with FODMAP sensitivities experience any kind of negative symptoms), intolerances depend largely on the quantity of food you eat. You can compare this phenomenon to any other food or drink. For example, drinking 5 gallons of water would most definitely kill you, but sticking to ½ or 1 gallon a day would keep you as healthy as a horse. The toxicity of the different things you ingest change as the quantities of those things changes as well. Thus, it is important to recognize that FODMAPs can wreak havoc on your system if you are not being aware of how much of each ingredient you are eating. We will go more in-depth on how to monitor your intake in later chapters and the recipe sections.

As I mentioned, FODMAPs themselves are not inherently bad, and scientists have found that most people who have a sensitivity to FODMAPs are, more likely than not, people with IBS. We will discuss IBS and its classic symptoms in detail in the next chapter, but before we do, it is important to recognize that different FODMAPs can affect different IBS sufferers in different ways.

Chapter 2: Benefits of the Low-FODMAP Diet

Who Should Follow the Low-FODMAP Diet?

Studies have shown that following a low-FODMAP diet can help alleviate the symptoms and extreme discomfort that IBS sufferers feel on a day-to-day basis. Though the diet is adapted for IBS sufferers, there are parts of the low-FODMAP diet that will also help reduce food-related discomfort for people who have mild gluten or dairy intolerances. I will delve more into the details about IBS in the following section.

If you have noticed that stress causes your bowel movements to change or increases the chances of you having stomach pain or cramps, you might want to try stress management as a treatment for IBS. However, if you have been practicing stress management techniques, but you don't see a definite decrease in the intensity and frequency of your IBS symptoms, I would highly suggest giving the low-FODMAP diet a chance. Although it is not for everyone, the low-FODMAP diet has shown in many studies that it helps reduce your daily symptoms and can help you return to a normal life when other methods are less effective.

To sum up, you should certainly give the low-FODMAP diet a go if you suffer from chronic and severe gut problems from IBS. I recommend you give this diet a sincere try, and I hope that you will see positive results!

What Is IBS?

IBS, or irritable bowel syndrome, is a condition that affects about 15% of the global population. It is also known by other more descriptive names, including irritable colon, spastic colitis, and mucous colitis. Although similarly named, IBS differs greatly from IBD, inflammatory bowel disease, which is an autoimmune condition that causes chronic inflammation and other issues along the entirety of the digestive tract. Aside from being painful and extremely disruptive, IBD can be life-threatening. Therefore, if you feel you may have IBD and not IBS, please see a doctor for your condition.

Classic IBS presents as a group of symptoms from the intestine, including abdominal pain or discomfort and changes in bowel habits, including frequency and form changes. To be diagnosed, these symptoms generally must last for at least 3 months and must occur at least 3 times a week. Although a good number of people with IBS experience on and off phases in their symptoms rather than persistent problems, symptoms can become chronic and much harder to control. A doctor may put you on the low-FODMAP as part of his or her diagnosis; if the diet seems to alleviate your symptoms, the doctor will feel more comfortable diagnosing you with IBS. If the diet does not seem to work for you, your doctor will likely test you for food allergies, infection, or celiac disease (gluten intolerance). If you have already been diagnosed with IBS, this book will help you follow the low-FODMAP diet, reduce uncomfortable gut symptoms, and potentially lose weight all at the same time!

Although IBS can affect all people, it most commonly occurs in individuals under the age of 50, and it is twice as common in women as it is in men. Women tend to experience worsened symptoms during or around the time they are menstruating. Some women may even confuse IBS symptoms with PMS. For example, IBS can cause lower back aches, more painful menstruation and menstrual cramps, and fatigue. Although all of these symptoms are, in some way, related to gut malfunction, there are several links between the severity of IBS and the progress of a woman through her childbearing years. It is important to reach out to your doctor if you feel that your symptoms are worsened during your menstrual period because it could be an indicator of another gynecological or gut-related problem. Although the exact relationship between a woman's digestive system and her reproductive system is still unclear, IBS is, for the most part, very similar between men and women.

IBS also seems to have a genetic component attached to it. If a family member has IBS and you begin to experience similar symptoms, it could be linked to the ways the nerves in your digestive tract function. IBS within a family can also point to risk factors in the common environment and lifestyles.

IBS can range from extremely mild to severe. Most people don't ever get treatment or see a doctor for their symptoms, but for individuals who experience frequent, severe symptoms, their quality of life can potentially become quite poor. IBS is an extremely unpredictable disorder, and the wide variety of symptoms can occur at any time and can sometimes have no causal link between anything you ate and the symptoms you experience. Doctors will generally diagnose an individual with IBS if two or more of the following characteristic symptoms are present as a long-term occurrence:

1. **Abdominal Pain and Cramping:** Abdominal Pain and Cramping: Abdominal pain cramping that becomes less severe or subsides entirely after a bowel movement is the most common symptom among all IBS sufferers. IBS cramping can be distinguished from other abdominal cramps you may experience because IBS cramps will always result in one of the following three scenarios: changes in stool consistency or color, changes in the frequency of bowel movements, and some pain relief after a bowel movement.

    We possess some helpful "good" bacteria in our gut that release signals to the brain and gut to help smooth bowel function to occur. Among IBS sufferers, these signals are lost or distorted and lead to irregular function of the muscles along the digestive tract. This leads to pain and muscle cramps in the middle and lower abdomen.

2. **Constipation:** Constipation: 50% of all IBS sufferers are afflicted with constipation-predominant IBS. Constipation or having less than three bowel movements a week is a common symptom of many ailments, but IBS-related constipation is different because it is generally accompanied by abdominal pain. Constipation is the result of nerve and gut signals that slow transit

of materials and stool throughout the digestive tract. When this happens, the bowel continues to absorb more and more water from the stool, making it even harder to pass. This condition is also characterized by the feeling of an incomplete or excessively strained bowel movement.

3. **Diarrhea:** Roughly 33% of all IBS sufferers are afflicted with diarrhea-predominant IBS. In this type of IBS, the stool is generally watery and tends to lead to very loose motions. Stools can even contain extra mucus from the digestive tract. Diarrhea-predominant IBS sufferers tend to experience an average of 12 bowel movements a week, and those movements can be sudden and extremely difficult to control. As with constipation-predominant IBS, this diarrhea is accompanied by pain that subsides after a bowel movement. Sudden-onset diarrhea can cause mental health repercussions as patients develop anxiety about their bowel movements and are held back from engaging in activities they are worried about.

4. **Alternating Constipation and Diarrhea:** Alternating Constipation and Diarrhea: Approximately 20% of IBS sufferers experience this type of mixed bowel movement routine. This type of IBS is again characterized by chronic and recurrent abdominal pain, but sufferers experience more intense and frequent symptoms. The phases of each type of bowel movement can last for days or weeks and can unpredictably

switch at any time, regardless of whether the individual's diet is consistent or suddenly changing.

5. **Gas and Bloating:** As we have seen, IBS causes a variety of digestive inconsistencies. This can lead to excess gas production in the gut, and the resulting uncomfortable bloating can become chronic. If gas, bloating, and pain are the most prevalent symptoms you experience with your IBS, a low-FODMAP diet is the most effective way to help reduce your discomfort.

Unlike IBD, scientists and doctors are still unable to pinpoint the exact cause of IBS. They have, however, identified some factors that do seem to play an important role in the symptoms many people experience.

1. **Miscommunication between the nervous system and gut:** The brain and gut work together to encourage smooth and regular bowel movements. If the signals between the brain and gut become uncoordinated, stool movement throughout the intestines can slow down or become excessively accelerated.

2. **Stress:** This is a major trigger for most IBS sufferers because it alters the way the nervous system performs daily functions. Since nervous system functionality and its ability to properly communicate is so important to regular gut function, stress generally worsens IBS symptoms. High-FODMAP foods can also worsen IBS

symptoms because of the extra gases they introduce to the body system. This generally leads to abdominal discomfort.

3. **Malfunction in the colon:** Sometimes, your colon can respond to different triggers by alternating between slow and spastic muscular movements that can damage tissue and cause painful cramping in your abdomen. Serotonin molecules can also collect in excessive amounts in the colon (most likely another effect of miscommunication between the brain and gut, as described above) and can lead to changes in muscular motility and resulting bowel movements. Finally, if you have mild celiac disease that is undiagnosed, you could be causing more harm to your intestines, which, in turn, could lead to a variety of IBS symptoms.

Since IBS is a chronic illness, treatments are geared toward long-term symptom management and not necessarily toward a concrete cure. IBS sufferers are, first and foremost, encouraged to discover and avoid their personal IBS triggers. Thus, as a general rule, individuals who are diagnosed with IBS are generally told to follow some form of the low-FODMAP diet and try and minimize the major stressors in their lives so they can experience a pain-free and more predictable life. Some doctors also recommend peppermint oil to help relax the bowel and types of therapy to help limit stress. If these "home-remedies" do not help make a significant positive impact on your quality of life as it relates to IBS, your doctor may look into putting you on prescription medication for your symptoms. In this book, we will be focusing on the benefits of the low-FODMAP diet and ways to follow it!

How Does the Low-FODMAP Diet Work?

Low-FODMAP should be restrictive only for a short amount of time to avoid deficiency in some essential nutrients. In the next chapter, we will delve more into how to maintain good nutrition while on the diet. For now, we will discuss how the diet works and the three steps that you should take to help the diet benefit you as much as possible. The low-FODMAP diet is generally divided into three phases where each has different limitations and goals. They are described below:

1. **Phase 1: Elimination.** This is the time when you will follow the low-FODMAP to a T and I encourage you to explore and follow all the recipes in this book during this phase. This phase will be the toughest one because you are limiting your high-FODMAP intake. This phase should last between 2-8 weeks depending on your body's response, and you should try not to stay on this restrictive diet for much longer than that. We will explain the reasoning behind this time frame in the next chapter.

   During this phase, you will eliminate all high-FODMAP foods from your diet and stick to a strict serving size for all ingredients and foods to ensure you are only eating foods in the low-FODMAP range. Remember that elimination is referring only to FODMAPs and you should not be eliminating entire food groups from your diet. Instead, you should aim to think of this diet as a substitution diet where you replace high-

FODMAP foods with low-FODMAP foods, like replacing an apple a day with an orange a day. This does eliminate high-FODMAP foods from your diet but still helps you maintain balance and nutrition.

2. **Phase 2: Reintroduction.** This phase should begin straight after the previous phase and should be planned while your elimination phase is still ongoing. It might be scary to start reintroducing foods back into your diet, particularly if the elimination phase considerably reduced your IBS symptoms. After 2-8 weeks of eliminating high-FODMAP foods and substituting low-FODMAP foods in their place, you should begin introducing reasonable amounts of high-FODMAP foods back into your diet, one subcategory at a time. This way, you give your body time to adjust to reintroduction and you will easily be able to tell which new foods are still intolerable to you.

As you are beginning to eat these foods again, the rest of your diet should remain low-FODMAP so that you can isolate the high-FODMAP foods you are eating. This phase can take up to 6-8 weeks, depending on how many foods you wish to try bringing back into your daily diet, and should be done methodically. Take your time with this phase, as it will be extremely helpful when you move onto the next phase and try to maintain a fully tolerable diet for yourself.

3. **Phase 3: Maintenance.** This is the "final" phase of the low-FODMAP diet, and it is when you have the freedom to personalize the diet so that you can maintain it long-term. You should only begin maintaining your ideal diet once you have fully identified and interpreted your trigger foods and the quantities you can tolerate other foods.

   This phase involves allowing your diet to go as close to normal as possible so that you are only controlling the intake of specific foods that trigger your IBS symptoms. It is important to note that a bowel afflicted with IBS can change unpredictably and cause you to become intolerant of foods you used to take well, and vice versa. If this happens, talk with your nutritionist and maybe try going through phase 2 again to identify your new triggers and tolerances. Eventually, you should be able to tolerate most high-FODMAP foods (again, in reasonable quantities) without setting off your IBS.

It is important to have a wide diet range, so please make sure to follow these three phases as best as you can. Our goal at the end of the low-FODMAP diet is to have hopefully expanded your diet and not further restricted it.

Benefits of the Low-FODMAP Diet

Research on the low-FODMAP diet has still not expanded to include all digestive disorders. However, one certain benefit of the low-FODMAP diet is a reduction in IBS symptoms that can disrupt your day-to-day life. You will hopefully see quick results when you begin the elimination phase and start the low-FODMAP diet. The benefits of this diet include decreased gas and bloating, more regular bowel movements, and less urgent bowel movements, all the way to better lifelong food tolerances and normalcy. You will also notice your bowel movements becoming more consistent in their form and color—gross, I know—but it is important to observe!

Studies have shown time and time again that 70% of IBS sufferers who followed the low-FODMAP diet in all its phases that we discussed previously saw significant and sustained improvement in their digestive symptoms. Those are excellent odds, and I hope you have a success story with this diet as well!

Chapter 3: Getting Started

Before You Start

Before you begin the low-FODMAP diet, try to meet with the doctor who diagnosed you with IBS, a primary care physician, a dietician, or a nutritionist. These professionals will help you become more confident with the remedy that you are going to committing to. This diet could be a major shift for you in terms of your eating and grocery-shopping habits. Thus, it is important to become actively conscious of the foods you are eating and much more aware of food labels, so you know exactly what ingredients you are putting in your body. Keep in mind that information about FODMAPs on food labels may be hard to come by. Still, you should try to do the best research so that you can get the most out of this diet.

Doing this will become especially important for you when you are trying to introduce some high-FODMAP foods back into your diet. The reintroduction period will be much easier if you know which meals and ingredients you have been eating and tolerating well. Make sure you also know a general outline of which foods are high, medium, and low in FODMAPs, and how changing your cooking methods and serving sizes can change how many FODMAPs you are eating. Finally, as you begin to get more comfortable with this new diet, try to continue testing which foods you can tolerate little by little outside of the low-FODMAP diet. This will help you when you are attempting to introduce foods back into your daily life.

Finally, before you start, I would encourage you to begin keeping a food log or journal. This will not be a task for you to count calories but to list down the ingredients you have eaten in a day and then log the IBS symptoms you feel in the next couple of days following that. In addition to logging that, I suggest you also journal a few sentences about how you felt immediately after each low-FODMAP meal you ate. Doing this every day will help you better track which foods you can tolerate and which foods, even some low-FODMAP foods, you need to eliminate from your diet for the time being. Finally, try to log other factors that could be contributing to your IBS symptoms. For example, if you are under a great deal of stress in your life or if you are on your menstrual cycle, write it down so you don't erroneously attribute all your symptoms to the foods you are eating.

Following the Diet and Maintaining Your Nutrition

Certain foods affect people with IBS more than other foods do. If you are already following a low-FODMAP diet and you feel as if your symptoms are only slightly improving, you may see a bigger difference if you cut down your intake of certain other "trigger" foods. It can sometimes become difficult to maintain proper nutrition while you are figuring out what your IBS triggers are. You may become more and more focused on making sure the foods you are eating are low-FODMAP and so, without realizing it, you might let a nutritional balance fly out the window. Although most low-FODMAP recipes help you stay nutritionally balanced, it is important to keep some important tips in mind. The following list contains some of the most common trigger foods for IBS symptoms and good alternatives you can choose to eat instead so that you still have a balanced diet:

1. **Gluten:** Many people with IBS can also be mildly gluten intolerant, though they will not experience an immune response to the protein, internal physiological changes, or potential malnutrition that comes with Celiac Disease. Instead of a full-blown allergy, gluten intolerance is simply a form of insensitivity and will generally present as diarrhea-predominant IBS. Choosing to isolate and discover how you respond to gluten in your diet may be worth your time, as limiting gluten intake or going on a gluten-free diet has been beneficial for many IBS sufferers.

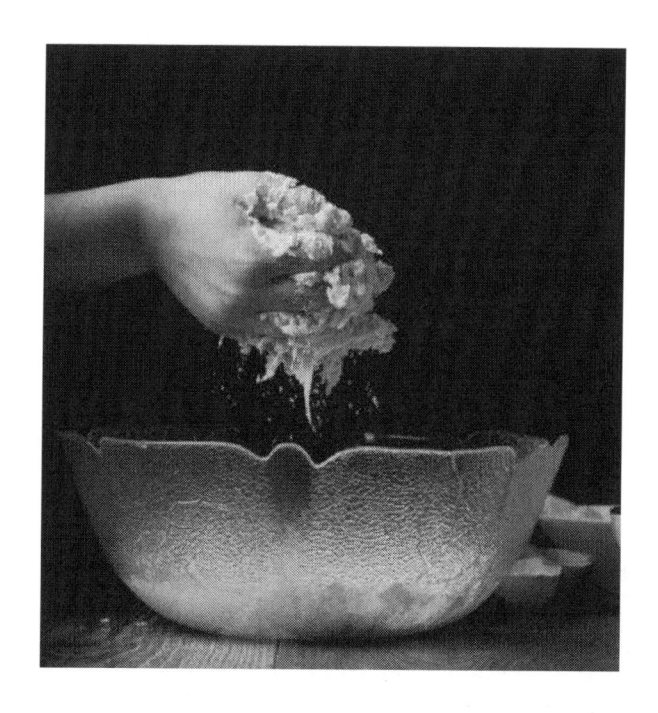

However, there are risks from going completely gluten-free if you are not actually gluten intolerant. You may become fiber-deficient, or you may experience deficiencies of other nutrients and vitamins that are heavily present in products that contain gluten. Please make sure to check with a nutritionist or your doctor before you adopt a gluten-free diet.

2. **Dairy:** Dairy products contain two potential red flags for people with IBS. First and foremost, dairy contains large amounts of lactose, a sugar that many people with IBS are intolerant of. Lactose is high-FODMAP and can result in some detrimental IBS symptoms. Some alternatives to lactose products include rice milk or soy-based cheeses and milk.

28

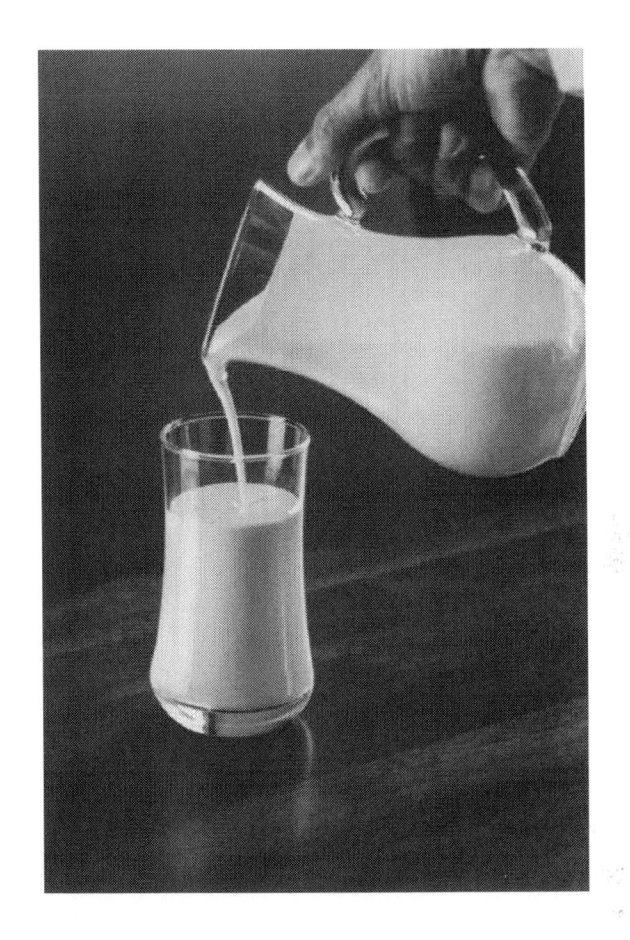

Dairy also contains a good amount of fat, which can encourage diarrhea production in your bowels. It is a good idea to begin consuming low or non-fat dairy products if you are experiencing diarrhea-predominant or alternating IBS. One major risk of reducing or eliminating your dairy intake is becoming deficient in calcium. Make sure to check in with a doctor and determine whether or not you need to be on a calcium supplement to restore a healthy calcium level.

3. **Insoluble Fibers:** Fiber is extremely important to a healthy diet because it helps to bulk up your meals and keep you full for longer. Fiber can even help relieve constipation and its symptoms. However, insoluble fibers can have detrimental effects on the gut of people who have IBS. Insoluble fiber passes through the gut very quickly and can worsen diarrhea symptoms, so many people with diarrhea are advised to stick to eating foods that have more soluble as opposed to insoluble fibers. Make sure you are still getting enough fiber in your diet to avoid becoming constipated. Foods like oatmeal, carrots, berries, and some legumes are good sources of soluble fibers, and these will help keep you full and hopefully alleviate some of your uncomfortable IBS symptoms.

4. **Caffeinated Drinks:** Caffeine is, in fact, a drug that can alter your digestive system functioning by accelerating some of its processes and can result in symptoms like diarrhea and other digestive irregularities. Most sodas and energy drinks contain caffeine and should be avoided not only for digestive health but for your overall health, as they contain many more harmful ingredients. The most common way that people consume caffeine is by drinking coffee, and this might be one of the most difficult things to begin cutting out of your diet. Although it may take some patience and hard work, removing or at least greatly decreasing your caffeine intake will have significant beneficial effects on your IBS symptoms.

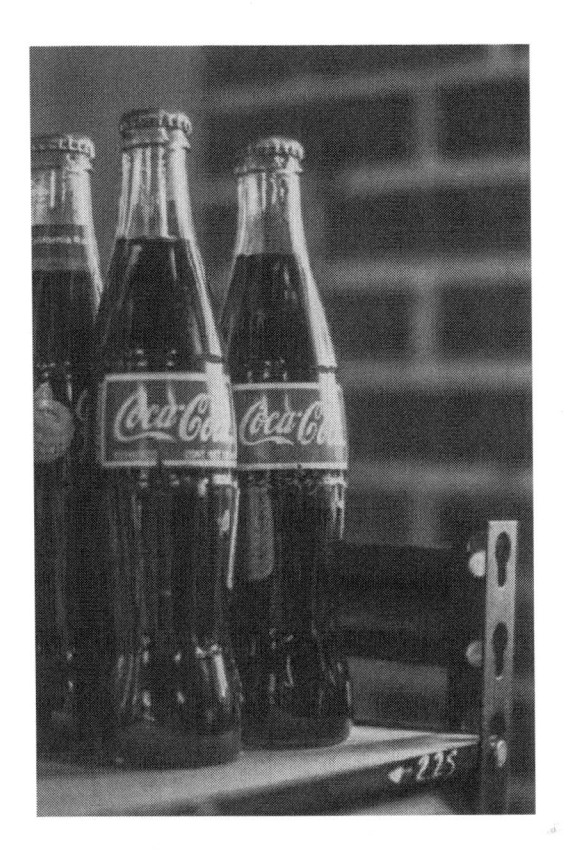

5. **Fried Foods:** As I mentioned above, consuming foods that have high-fat content can be harmful to people who experience IBS symptoms. Although fried foods like French fries, chicken strips, and even potato chips are common staples around the world, it is important to heavily reduce your intake of these items. Doing so will not only help improve your overall health but will also help minimize the discomfort of diarrhea and other IBS symptoms. If you are still looking to change up some of the foods you eat, consider grilling or

baking your ingredients as a healthier and more low-FODMAP friendly alternative.

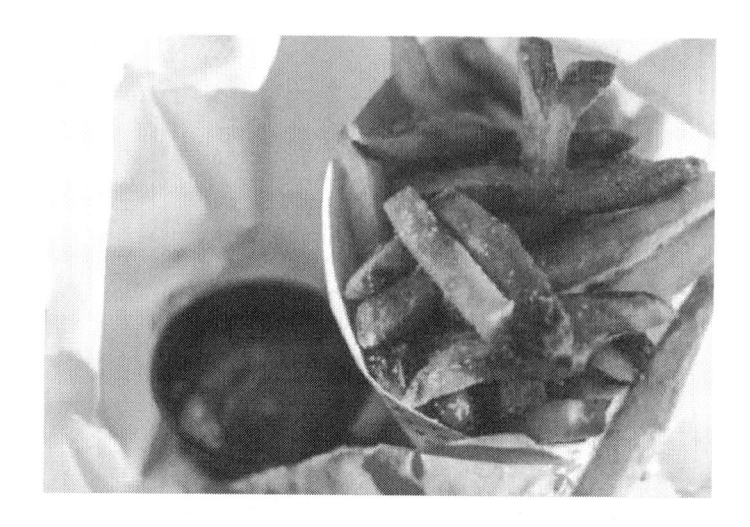

6. **Sugar-Free Sweeteners:** Although the term sugar-free can sound like a positive thing, it is full of hidden ingredients that are not only harmful to overall health but also, and most especially, to your IBS. These sugar-free sweeteners make up an entire FODMAP category on their own—they are known as polyols or sugar alcohols and contain ingredients like acesulfame potassium, aspartame, and sucralose. These ingredients are especially difficult to absorb in the bowels of people who suffer from IBS, so they are free to wreak havoc on your gut and bowel movements. These sweeteners are hidden in many items that are advertised as sugarless, including diet sodas and drinks, candies and gum, and even mouthwash. Please be cautious and read the labels of any sugary items you choose to buy, so you don't accidentally end up with a preventable IBS flare-up.

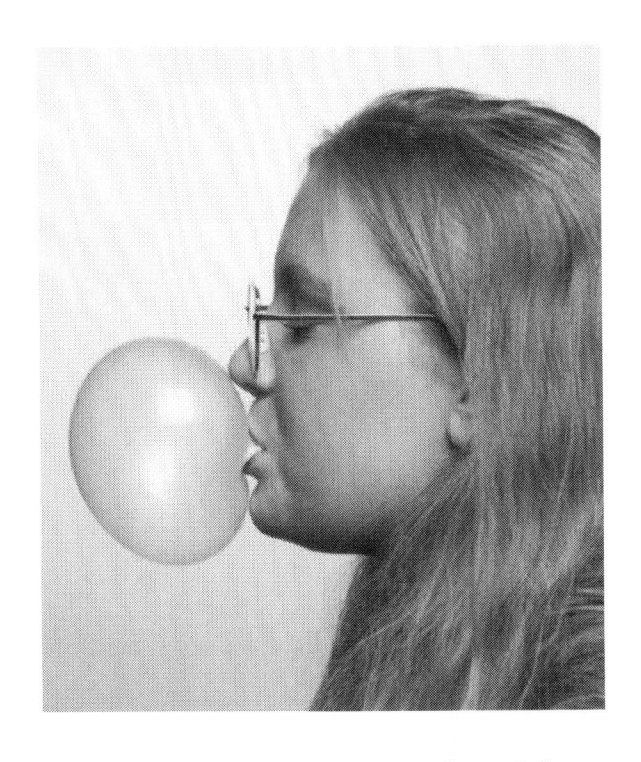

7. **Beans and Legumes:** Even though beans and legumes have a great number of health and nutritional benefits associated with them, they are naturally high in oligos and fructans and can be tricky to fit in a low-FODMAP diet. Beans tend to cause gas and bloating in the lower abdomen and can even bulk up stool and make bowel movements difficult to pass for some people. Still, there are ways to incorporate beans and legumes into a good low-FODMAP diet. For example, beans and legumes that have been canned or boiled can be lower in FODMAPs because the oglios from the products will leach out into the water that you drain out. Thus, a good cooking

method is imperative to keeping beans and lentils in your day-to-day low-FODMAP diet.

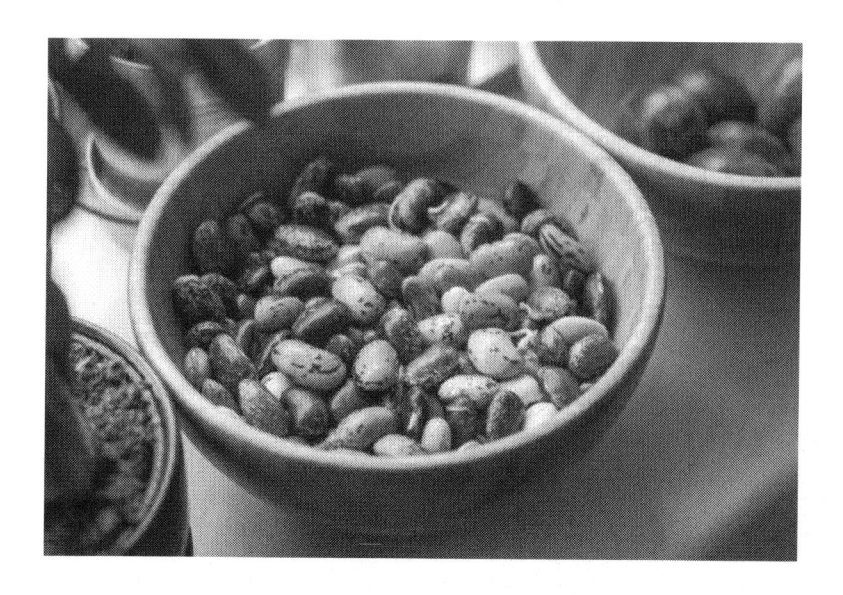

8. **Processed Foods:** The additives and preservatives in processed foods can cause significant flare-ups in people who suffer from IBS. These products can contain large quantities of one, if not more, of the FODMAPs and thus, will negatively affect your gut. Foods like chips, cookies, some frozen meals, and even some types of cereals and granola bars can contain high amounts of sugar and have high-fat content. Candies and chocolates can also contain caffeine, and as we learned earlier, excess fat and caffeine intake can contribute largely to worsened symptoms in diarrhea-predominant IBS. Some people have found that eating small amounts of vegan chocolate can be more tolerable, but this should be done with caution. I urge you to stay far

away from processed foods, not only while you are actively following the low-FODMAP diet but also after your diet relaxes a little bit to help reduce extra symptoms.

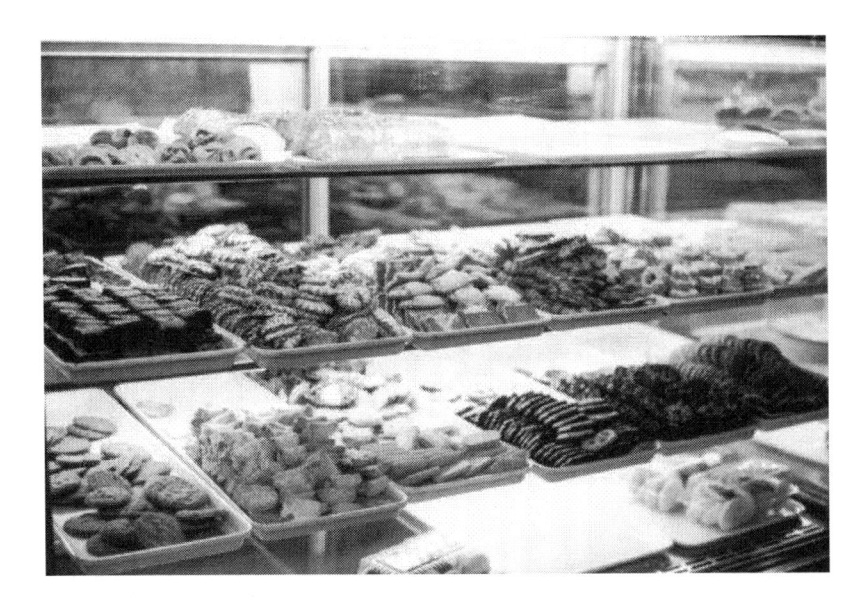

It is important to remember that each body is different and that each type of IBS can present very differently across a population. For that reason, you should take the time to figure out the needs and triggers of your own body so that you can create a diet that works best for you. The low-FODMAP diet is a great starting place, but you should feel free to adapt the guidelines (within reason) and maybe even check in with a dietician or nutritionist to find a diet that fully benefits your digestion and body function.

Things to Avoid

One of the most important things to remember when you begin to follow the low-FODMAP diet is that it is not a no-FODMAP diet, and it certainly should not become a lifetime diet. Certain foods that contain FODMAPs like fructans are beneficial for our naturally present gut bacteria. Thus, totally eliminating FODMAPs from your diet for months can cause more problems than it will solve.

Instead, begin by eliminating high-FODMAP foods and follow the diet as best as you can for a short period (2-6 weeks) and then check in with a nutritionist or your doctor to assess the effects it has had on your IBS symptoms. Do not continue the diet for months and months without making observations and measurements about how the diet is helping you. It is important to check in with a professional after about 8 weeks of following the diet to make sure it is doing what it is supposed to and that you are maintaining a nutritionally adequate diet. After the initial period of following a stricter low-FODMAP diet, your nutritionist will be able to help you identify the most problematic FODMAPs for your body. You will be able to reintroduce FODMAPs back into your diet slowly and only control the intake of the ones that are most sensitive to you. Thus, it is important to avoid starting this diet on your own without any professional guidance. Although this book is full of information about the low-FODMAP diet, IBS, and recipes you can use, it is not a one-size-fits-all solution to gut problems.

The front cover of this book advertises that the low-FODMAP diet will not only help your gut problems subside but will also help you lose weight. I want to make clear that this book is not telling you that simply eating meals made from the recipes listed in this book will make you lose hard weight. The low-FODMAP diet can instead help you lose water weight that the FODMAPs in your system have been retaining for so long. Additionally, following a low-FODMAP diet will help your gut "deflate" because the bacteria in your gut will not be producing as many harmful gas bubbles. This will help you feel less bloated and will, in turn, make you look slimmer. Additionally, if you have normally been eating meals that go way beyond recommended serving sizes, you may begin to lose weight when you stick to the ingredient serving sizes and meal portions that are listed in the recipes in this book. Still, I want to emphasize that the low-FODMAP diet has benefits that go far beyond simple weight loss, and you should not follow this diet solely to lose weight. The low-FODMAP diet is intended to help alleviate the symptoms individuals who suffer from IBS experience. Weight loss is an added but not a guaranteed bonus to following this diet.

Finally, remember that this diet is not meant to limit your calorie intake. It is only meant to help alleviate your gastrointestinal problems by limiting the amount of high-FODMAP foods you ingest. Thus, having a "cheat day" is not encouraged while you are following this diet. A single cheat day with a weight loss diet will not do you much harm and will not set you back too far. However, a cheat day with this diet, especially as your body is beginning to become used to more tolerable foods, could cause an increase in the intensity and frequency of your IBS symptoms. Since IBS is so unpredictable, it is hard to say how long your body might experience the setbacks from a single cheat day. The low-FODMAP diet is easily adaptable, and you will be able to eat plenty of pleasurable foods. Thus, we encourage you to try your best to stick to the diet for as long as you have been guided to do so. This will help alleviate your symptoms and get results on a much quicker timeline.

Example Shopping List

Some foods are naturally low-FODMAP foods, but others are only low-FODMAP in specific quantities. This basic example of a grocery shopping list does not offer suggested serving sizes, so please make sure to check how much of each food you should be eating if you are concerned. Some suggested serving sizes and low-FODMAP shopping tips are listed for the ingredients from the recipes in the following chapters. This is a far more general list.

Protein:
- Canned tuna and salmon
- Firm tofu
- Beef
- Chicken
- Lamb
- Egg
- Pork

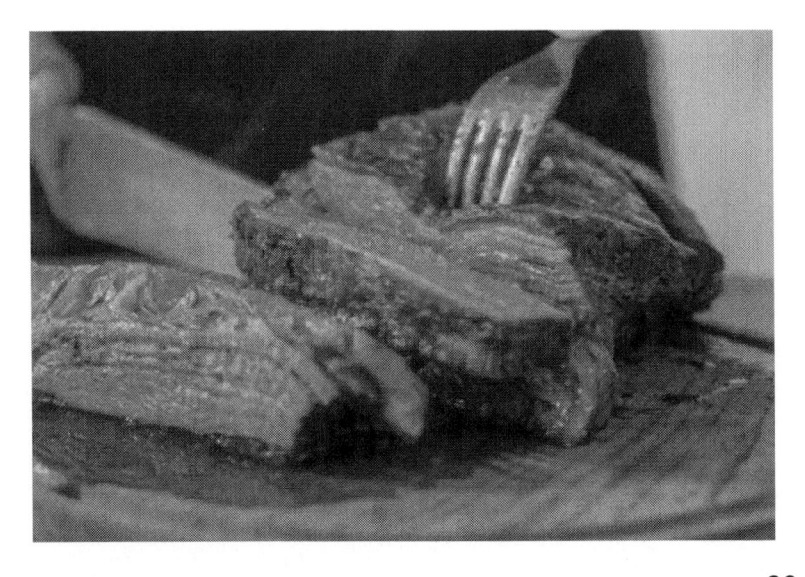

Grains:
- Gluten-free pasta
- Rice
- Quinoa
- Oats
- Oat bran
- Rice bran

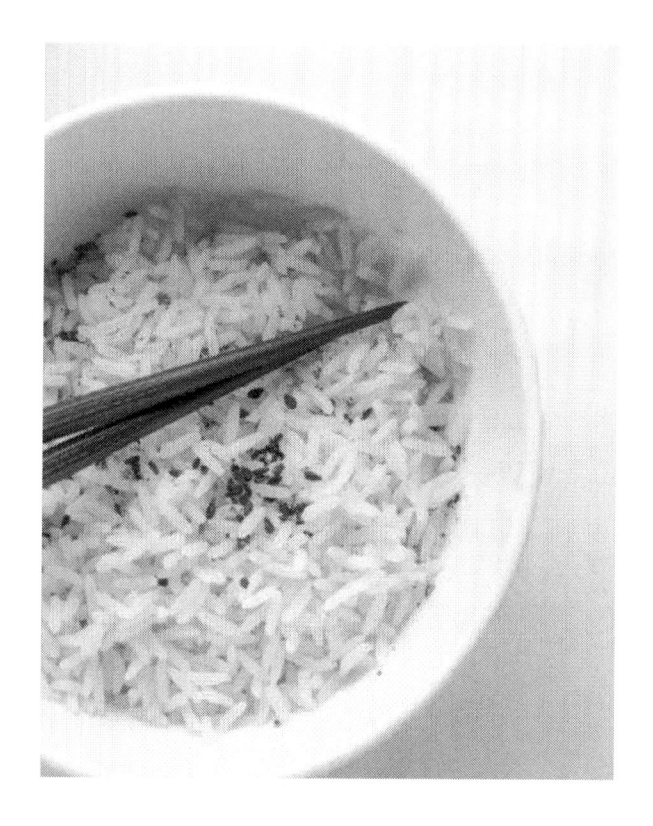

Milk:
- Canned coconut milk
- Almond milk
- Hemp milk
- Rice milk

- Lactose-free milk

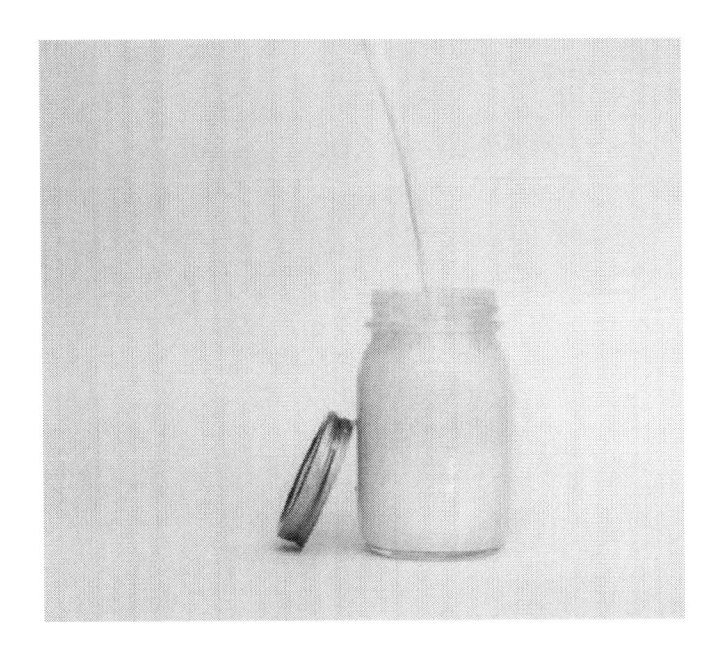

Cheeses:
- Mozzarella cheese
- Parmesan cheese
- Feta cheese
- Colby cheese
- Low fat cream cheese
- Cheddar cheese
- Low fat cottage cheese
- Brie cheese
- Swiss cheese
- Goat cheese

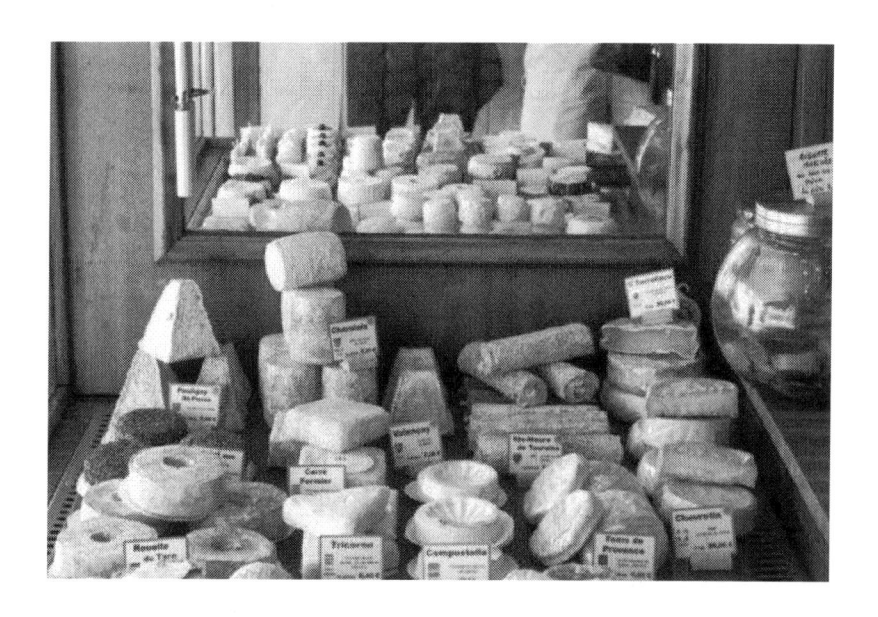

Fruits
- Small, firm bananas
- Blueberries, raspberries, strawberries
- Avocado
- Cantaloupe or honeydew melons
- grapes
- Clementines and oranges
- Pineapple
- Kiwifruit

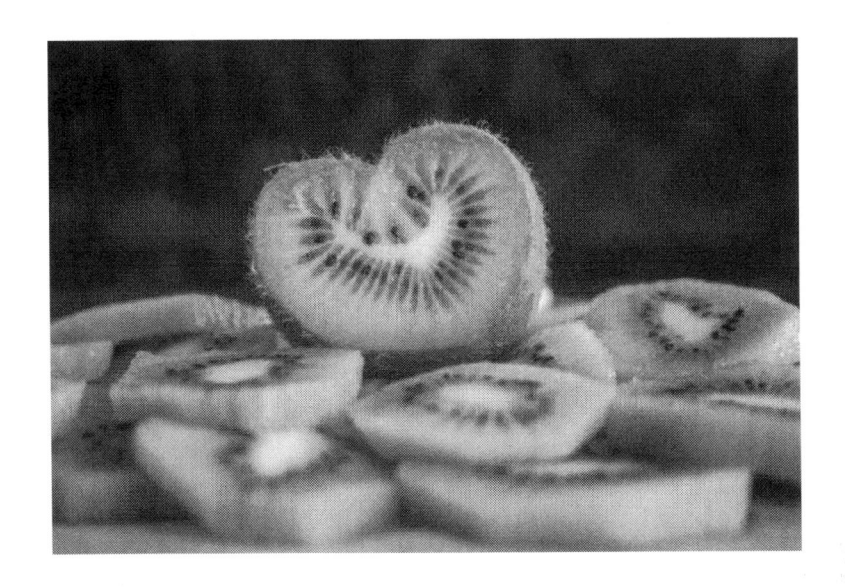

Vegetables
- Kale, Arugula, Spinach, Lettuce
- Zucchini
- Scallions (green part only)
- Bell Peppers
- Broccoli
- Red cabbage
- Leeks (green leaves only)
- Capers
- Green Beans
- White potatoes
- Sweet potatoes
- Carrots
- Summer squash
- Celery

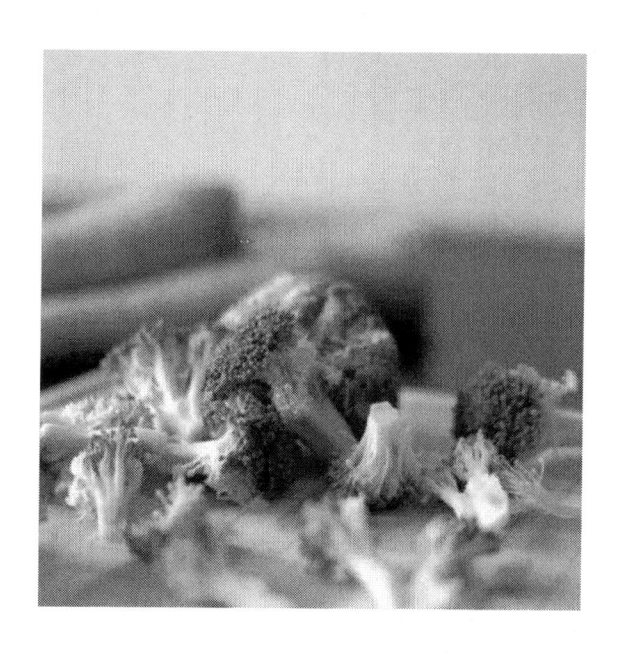

Chapter 4: Breakfast Recipes

Strawberry Chia Pudding

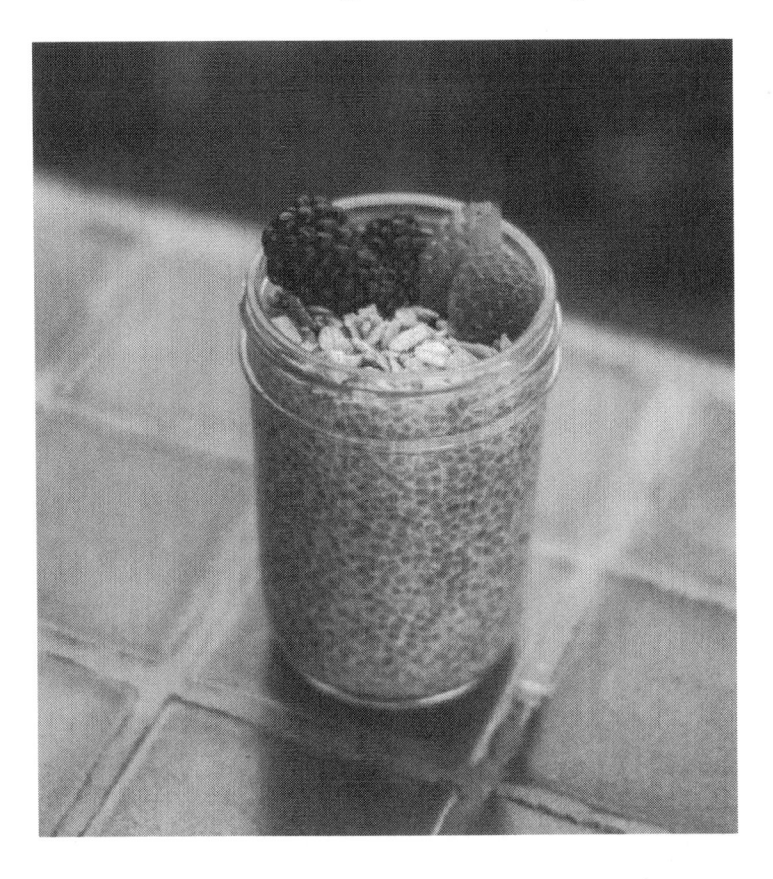

This is the ideal food for someone who needs a pre-made breakfast ready to grab and go in the morning. If you make this pudding at night, it will have thickened and will be ready for you in the morning! Chia seeds help make this meal fiber-rich while keeping the FODMAP count low so your gut can feel good. Still, chia seeds are a source of fiber, and you should be cautious when introducing them to your diet. The serving size listed below shouldn't give you any problems. This recipe will take only about 5 minutes to prepare and will give you 4 servings (1 serving is the low-FODMAP serving).

What You Will Need:
- 1 blender or food processor
- 1 bowl and enough plastic wrap to cover it
- 2 cups of almond milk
- 2 tbsp pure maple syrup
- 1 small basket of strawberries
- ½ cup chia pudding
- 1 handful of other low-FODMAP fruits

Low-FODMAP Shopping Tips:
- Choose a pure maple syrup rather than maple-flavored syrup because that could contain high-FODMAP ingredients.
- Check the example list in chapter 3 for examples of low-FODMAP fruits that you could use to top your chia seed pudding. Take care not to exceed more than a handle of whichever fruit you choose. You can also alter this recipe and add a small handful of low-FODMAP seeds or nuts.

Method:
1. Begin by adding your strawberries into your blender and then pour in all of your almond milk. Blend these two ingredients until they fully combine into a homogenous mixture.

2. Pour this mixture out of the blender and into your bowl. Stir in your maple syrup fully and then add in your chia seeds.

3. At this point, your pudding is already done! Cover the bowl with the pudding-to-be tightly with plastic wrap or film and set the bowl in the refrigerator. This soaking and cooling time will allow the chia seeds to expand which causes the milk mixture to thicken into the perfect pudding, so it is best if you let it sit in the fridge for a few hours. If you want breakfast ready for the morning, let it rest in the fridge overnight.

4. After the fridge time, pull the plastic wrap and top your pudding with your choice of low-FODMAP fruits! Enjoy!

Breakfast Smoothie

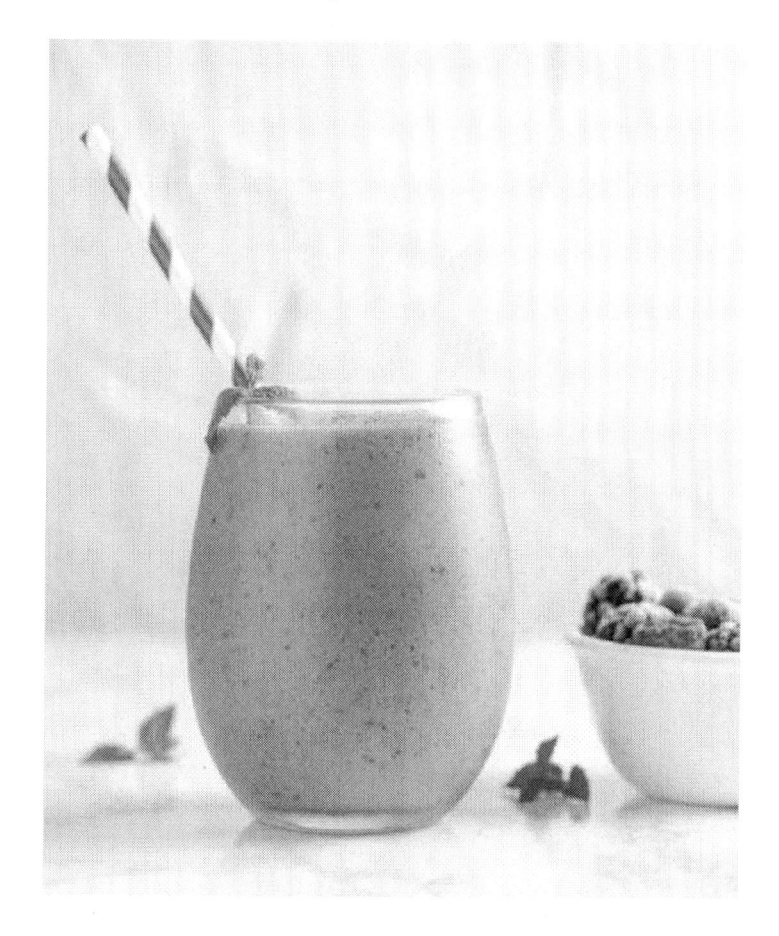

Smoothies can easily become high in FODMAPs if you include products like milk (lactose) or excess fruit quantities (fructose). However, it is easy to adapt your smoothies to be delicious while keeping your FODMAP ingestion low! This recipe is ideal for the elimination phase of your diet.

What You'll Need
- 1 serving of a low-FODMAP fruit

- o   Based on the flavor you desire
- o   Examples include: 1 medium-sized banana, 10 raspberries, 20 blueberries, 2 small kiwis, and 20 medium-sized strawberries.
- Protein Item
    - o   Examples include: 1–2 tbsp peanut butter, 1 tbsp tahini (sesame product), 1 tbsp almond butter *or* protein powder such as 2 tbsp pea protein, whey protein **isolate,** or brown rice protein
- Leafy Greens (Optional)
    - o   Examples Include: ½ cup kale or spinach or ½ cup cucumber peeled
- Fiber Item (Optional: if fiber is newer in your diet, make sure to add it in gradually)
    - o   Examples Include ¼ cup uncooked oats, 2 tbsp chia seeds, or 1 tbsp flax seeds.

Method:

This is the easiest part! Put all your ingredients into a blender of your choice and mix together until you've created a homogenous mixture with the consistency you desire. You can thin out your smoothie by adding in some water or thicken it by blending in some ice cubes. Keep in mind that smoothies are notorious for introducing too much fruit into your diet, so make sure to stick to the recommended serving sizes. Pour into a glass and enjoy!

Spinach and Salmon Omelette

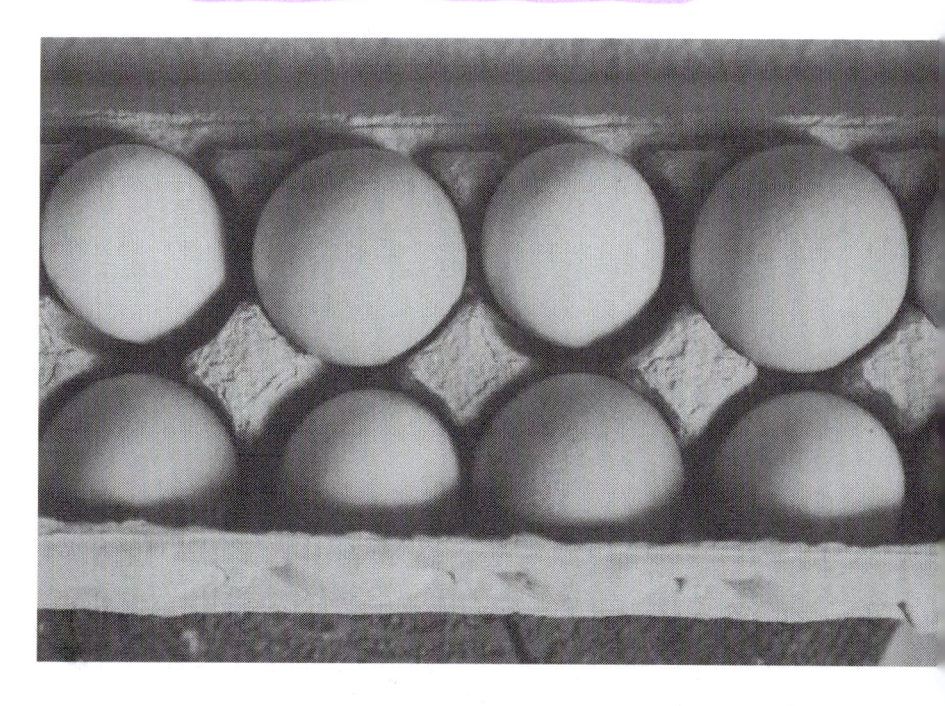

This tasty dish is perfect for a lazy breakfast date for two and can also become a quick lunch! The salmon and spinach add a great flavor to your omelet, and the cherry tomato topping brings all the flavors together. The omelet itself is so easy to throw together—it takes only 15 minutes to cook and yields 2 servings.

What You Will Need:
- 1 large frying pan
- 1 small mixing bowl
- 1 medium frying pan
- 8 cherry tomatoes
- 6 large eggs
- 2 cups of spinach
- 210 g of canned plain pink salmon

- Salt and pepper
- ⅛ tsp of paprika
- 2 tbsp of fresh parsley
- 1 and ½ tbsp of a low-FODMAP milk
- 2 tsp of sunflower, canola, OR rice bran oil (natural oil)
- 2 tsp of sesame oil

Low-FODMAP Shopping Tips:
- Make sure the canned salmon you buy is plain and contains no onions or garlic. An alternative to canned salmon is to buy fresh and cook it before integrating it into this recipe.

Method:
1. In your mixing bowl, combine the eggs and low-FODMAP milk until they are well mixed. Add salt and pepper to season the mixture.

2. Place your medium frying pan over medium-high heat, add some of your natural oil to the pan, and pour your egg mixture in. Sprinkle a light amount of paprika over the top of the omelet and cook until it is firm. If the top of the omelet does not cook well, you can flip it over and cook for another minute in the pan. Mind the heat while you cook, as the omelet can easily burn if left on too high for too long.

3. As the omelet is cooking, completely drain the salmon from the can and mix it with parsley and sesame oil in a small mixing bowl, dusting with some pepper and salt. Wash and shred your

spinach and cut in half your cherry tomatoes. Now, place your large frying pan over medium heat, and cook your salmon mixture until it is evenly heated throughout. When almost done cooking, add in your spinach and cook until the leaves wilt.

4. Plate your omelet, and pour your salmon and spinach mixture over it. Finally, top the dish with your halved cherry tomatoes and some black pepper. Enjoy!

Vegetable Omelet or Scramble

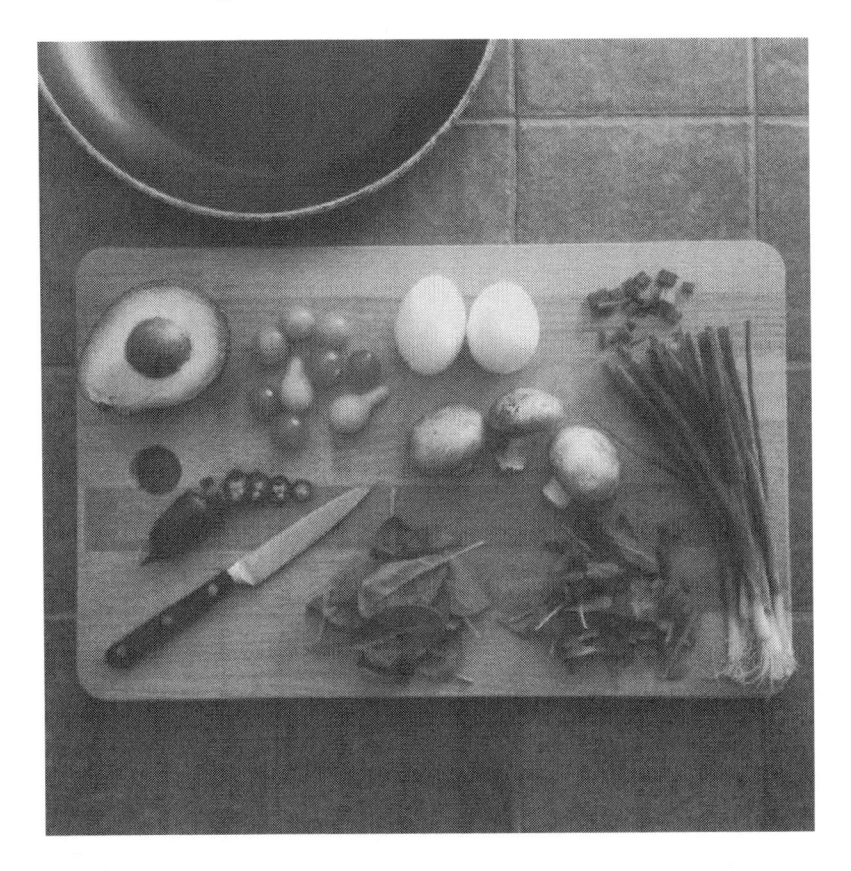

Eggs are a perfect low-FODMAP ingredient that is easy to prepare and provides a wide range of versatility! For example, if it is difficult to tolerate whole eggs, try experimenting with only using egg whites or pairing your eggs with different ingredients to help calm your IBS symptoms. Although this recipe includes only low-FODMAP veggies, try to limit your veggie count to 1 cup total so as not to overdo your veggie serving.

Low-FODMAP Veggies You Can Include:
- 1 cup of Bok choy

- ½ cup of Red and green bell peppers
- ½ cup of Kale
- ½ cup of Zucchini
- 1 small Tomato
- 1 bunch of Spring onion/scallion - *green part only*
- ¾ cup of broccoli florets
- 1 cup of spinach

Method:
Choose your veggies and chop them up into small cuts so that they integrate nicely into your eggs. Use 1–3 eggs (try to avoid using multiple yolks) and begin preparing them as you normally would—omelet or scrambled style. Before the eggs finish cooking, add in your veggies. Finish cooking as normal, and you have prepared the perfect Low-FODMAP breakfast that is also high in protein! You can even pair this dish with a side of roasted potatoes. Plate and enjoy!

Chocolate Porridge

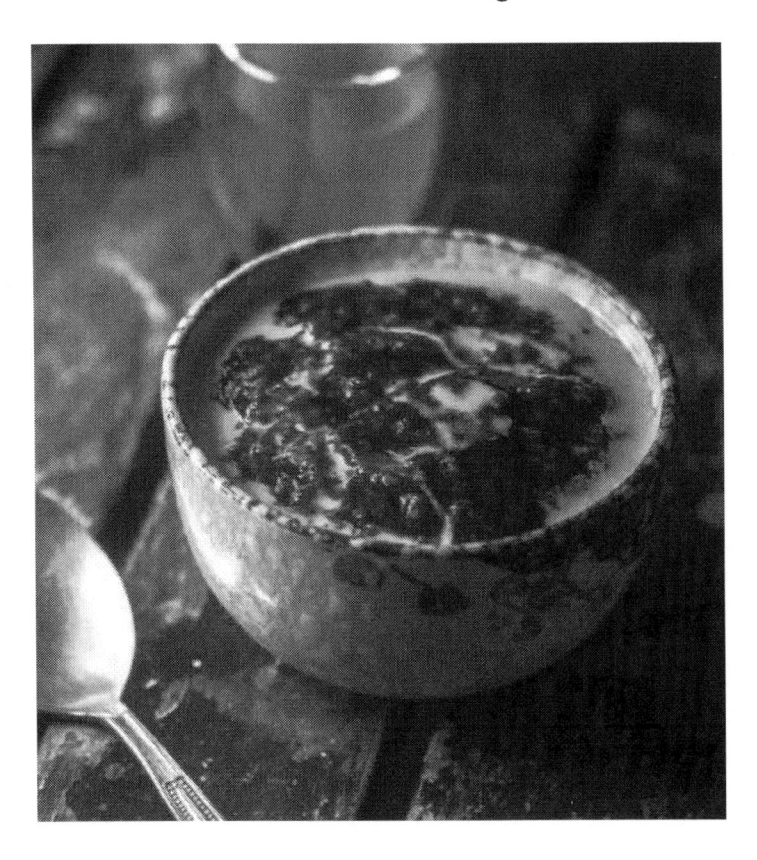

This chocolate porridge is a great way to enjoy the classic strawberries and chocolate combination while still getting a nutritious and filling meal in your system. This recipe uses cocoa powder rather than actual chocolate to limit the amount of FODMAPs and the amount of other unnecessary ingredients. As an alternative, you can top the porridge with a low-FODMAP yogurt and mint leaves to create a fresh twist! This recipe takes not more than 10 minutes total for preparation and cooking time and yields a full bowl of delicious chocolate oatmeal.

What You Will Need:
- 1 saucepan
- 20 g of chopped pecans
- 125 g of chopped strawberries
- ⅓ cup of rolled oats
- 1 tsp of table sugar
- 1 and ½ tsp of cocoa powder
- 1 cup of almond milk unsweetened

Low-FODMAP Shopping Tips:
- All the ingredients used in this recipe are low-FODMAP, provided you stick to the serving sizes we have listed above. If you want to be extra cautious with the oats, you can substitute rolled quinoa in place of rolled oats. If you want to be extra cautious with the milk, you can choose lactose-free milk in place of unsweetened almond milk.
- Choose pure cocoa powder to make sure it contains no other ingredients besides cocoa.

Method:
1. Begin by adding the oats and low-FODMAP milk to a small saucepan that is over medium heat. Stir in the table sugar and cocoa powder.

2. Let the oats mixture come to a bubble, then lower the heat, and let the oats cook for about 5 minutes until they reach the consistency you desire. Continue to stir the oatmeal as it is cooking to help prevent it from sticking to the pot.

3. Serve the porridge in a bowl, top it with strawberries and pecans, and enjoy your breakfast!

Breakfast Wrap

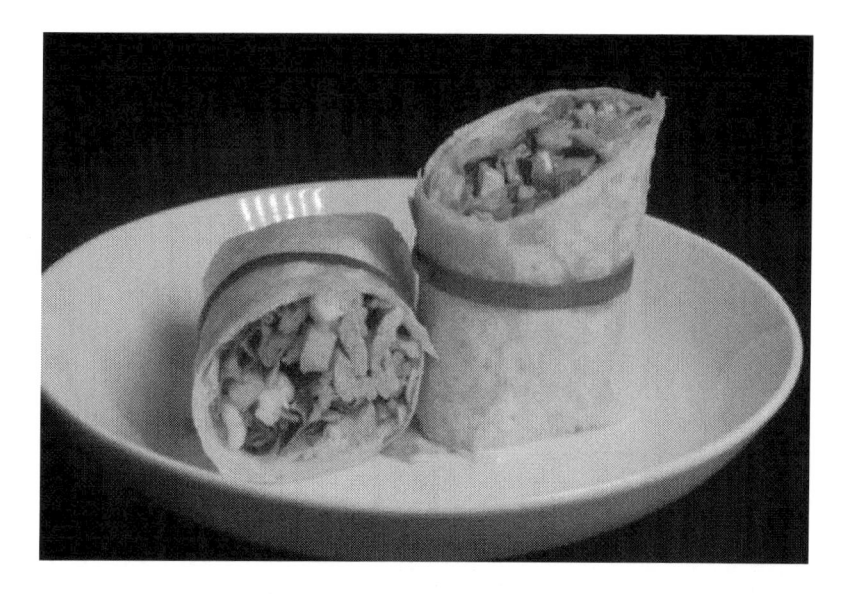

Wraps are another way to introduce versatility into your diet and are a great way to start your day! Since we are going for low-FODMAP diets, make sure to start your wrap with a gluten-free base, such as a corn tortilla.

Ideas for the Wrap Filling:
- ½ cup of spinach
- Scrambled eggs (try only egg whites if you are sensitive to whole eggs)
- ½ cup of bell peppers
- 1 medium tomato
- Potatoes
- 1-2 slices of low-FODMAP cheese (e.g., cheddar)
- ⅛ of the whole avocado
- 1 bunch of green onions/scallions (only use green part)

Method:
Select the ingredients you would like to include in your wrap and prepare them in any way you would like. For example, you can either roast/sauté your veggies or simply include them raw. Once you have the ingredients you like, simply wrap up the cooked tortilla around the filling and you have a wholesome breakfast. Enjoy!

Banana Pancakes

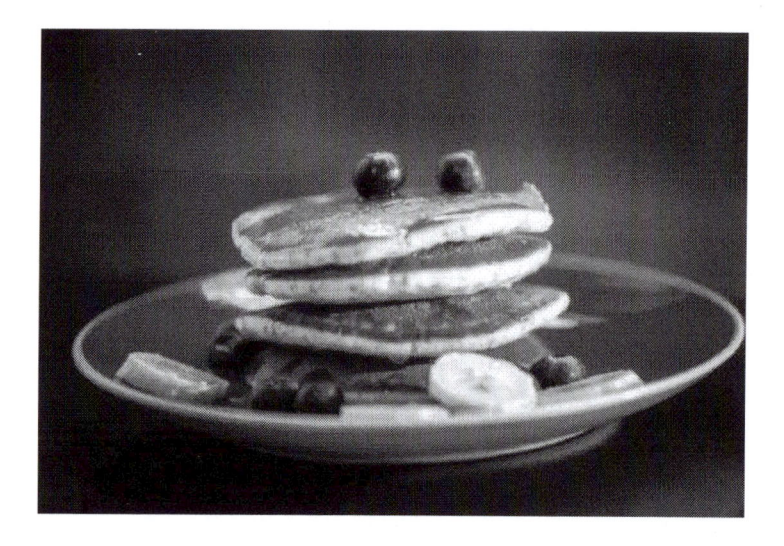

These mini pancakes are a nutritious and delicious way to start your day because it is like eating banana bread in pancake form! Although these pancakes are tasty and filling on their own, try pairing them with a low-FODMAP fruit and yogurt suggested below for some extra flavors and textures. This recipe will take you about 20 minutes to prepare and will leave you with 8 delicious mini pancakes to share with a friend!

What You Will Need:
- 1 large mixing bowl
- 1 large frying pan
- 2 firm bananas
- 10 blueberries
- 2 large eggs
- 6 tbsp of lactose-free yogurt (or coconut yogurt)
- 2 tbsp of gluten-free all-purpose flour
- 3 tbsp of olive oil spread OR dairy-free butter

- Powdered sugar
- ¼ tsp of baking powder
- ½ tsp of ground cinnamon
- ¼ tsp of ground nutmeg
- 1 pinch of salt
- 1 tbsp of brown sugar (tightly packed)

Low-FODMAP Shopping Tips:
- Choose low-FODMAP yogurt that is free of inulin, lactose, agave syrup, fruit juice, honey, fructose, high-fructose corn syrup, and high-FODMAP fruits.
- Choose a pure gluten-free flour that contains no chickpea/garbanzo flour, coconut flour, soy flour, lentil flour, amaranth flour, or lupin flour.
- Choose common bananas that are firm and still very slightly green. Once the bananas ripen and begin to develop spots, they become high-FODMAP.

Method:
1. Begin by peeling the bananas and mashing them in a large mixing bowl. Add in the eggs and whisk in the bananas. Combine the salt, cinnamon, gluten-free flour, nutmeg, brown sugar, and baking powder with the bananas, and make sure to mix well.

2. Add a tablespoon of your dairy-free spread to a frying pan as it heats up on a medium flame. Start cooking the pancakes by scooping about 3 tbsp of batter into the pan, one at a time. Once you see

bubbles beginning to form on the top surface of the pancake, flip and allow it to cook until both sides are golden brown. Continue cooking the pancakes until you are out of batter on consistent heat and adding more dairy-free spread if necessary.

3. Serve the pancakes in a stack with your yogurt and berries. Sprinkle powdered sugar on top of the pancakes if you desire. Enjoy!

Green Smoothie

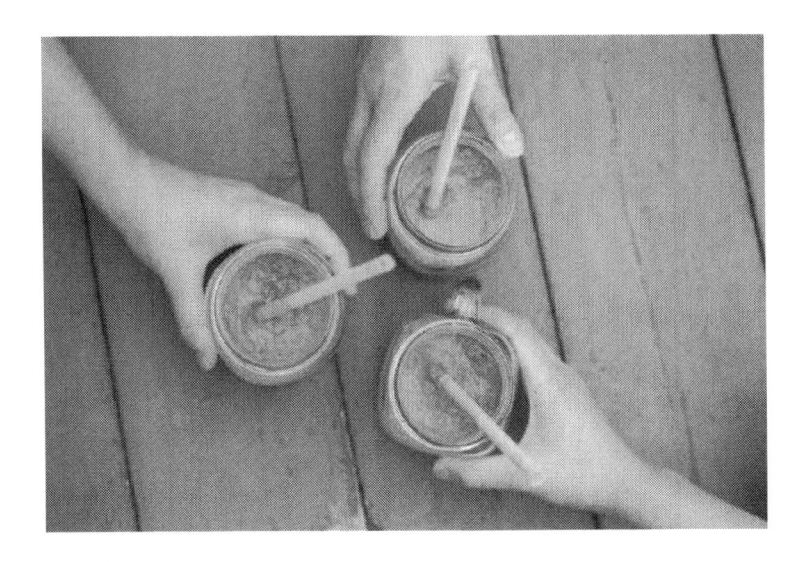

This smoothie is the perfect blend of sweet and tart and will be an energizing way to start your day! Everything used in this recipe is low-FODMAP and still, this smoothie manages to have healthy amounts of fiber and vitamins A and C. Your nutrition will certainly not be compromised with this smoothie! There are many ways to personalize this recipe, so keep reading for ways you can change it up and make it your own. Don't worry; you will not get any bitter flavors that will leave you wondering why you mixed greens into a fruit blend, to begin with. Two glasses of this smoothie (serving size is 1) only take about 5 minutes to whip and will leave you obsessed with your new breakfast option.

What You Will Need:
- 1 blender or food processor
- Approx. 8 inches of an English cucumber
- 1 cup of green grapes (try for seedless grapes)

- 1 whole kiwi
- 1-2 2 cups of ice cubes
- 2 cups of baby spinach (you can use Lacinato Kale leaves for a more intense flavor)

Method:
1. Begin by figuring out which end of your blender the blade is on. We want to put the grapes either first or last, depending on the blade position so that they get the blending process started smoothly.

2. Next, peel your kiwi and cut it into large chunks. Leave the English cucumber unpeeled, and cut that into chunks as well, a little smaller this time. If you are using kale leaves rather than baby spinach, make sure the kale is properly washed, stemmed, and roughly chopped.

3. Now, add all your ingredients, except the ice cubes, to the blender, making sure to keep the grapes closest to the blade. Pulse your blender on and off a few times to get the ingredients to blend slightly, and then blend at high speed until you see a green, homogeneous mixture in your blender. There should be no chunks or pieces of grated leaves in there.

4. Once the mixture is ready, add a few ice cubes at a time and blend everything together until the smoothie becomes a little frosty. You can continue adding ice if you desire. It will help thicken the smoothie and cool your drink.

5. Pour into a glass and drink before the ingredients begin to separate. Enjoy!

In this recipe, we used grapes and kiwi because they can offer either sweet or tangy flavors, depending on how ripe they are. Since the ripeness does not change the FODMAP count in either fruit, you are at liberty to choose how ripe you would like your fruits to be, particularly kiwi. We also recommend that first-time green smoothie drinkers use baby spinach instead of kale. Spinach has a much milder flavor, whereas kale offers a bold flavor that some people can find overwhelming if they are not used to it. Finally, feel free to add in a handful of low-FODMAP berries into this smoothie as long as you stay within the recommended FODMAP serving sizes. Enjoy your customizable smoothie!

French Toast with Banana and Pecans

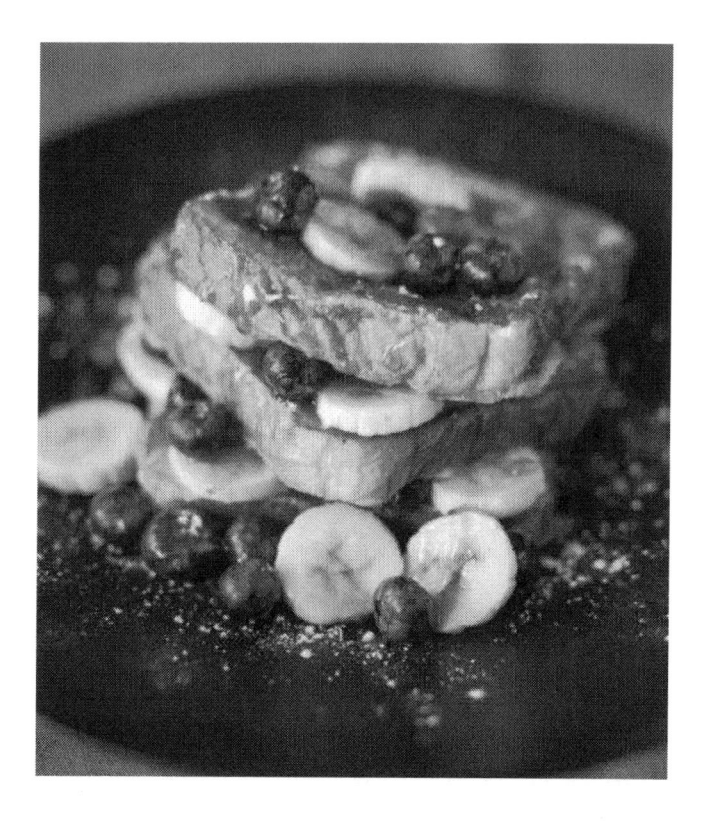

This recipe is a healthy and delicious way to change the normal breakfast routine that you have been following. It is the perfect morning pick-me-up in the middle of the week! If you are on a nut-free diet for whatever reason, you can change this recipe to include toasted pumpkin or sunflower seeds instead. The recipe below takes only 10 minutes to make and will yield 2 slices or 1 serving of an amazing low-FODMAP French toast breakfast!

What You Will Need:
- 1 large frying pan
- 1 wide, flat bowl

- 1 egg
- 2 slices of a low-FODMAP bread
- Half a banana
- ½ tbsp olive oil spread or dairy-free butter
- 1 tsp of ground cinnamon
- 2 tsp of maple syrup pure
- 2 tbsp of crumbled pecans (OR sunflower/pumpkin seeds)

Low-FODMAP Shopping Tips:
- Choose a pure maple syrup rather than maple-flavored syrup because that could contain high-FODMAP ingredients.
- Buy low-FODMAP bread that contains no chickpea/garbanzo flour, coconut flour, soy flour, amaranth flour, or lupin flour. Also, try to avoid ingredients like concentrated fruit juices, pear juice, apple juice, inulin, apple fiber, high-fructose corn syrup, or honey. Wheat sourdough bread can be a good low-FODMAP option
- Choose common bananas that are firm and still very slightly green. Once the bananas ripen and become to develop spots, they become high-FODMAP.

Method:
1. Begin to heat your large frying pan over medium heat. As it heats up, add in your dairy-free butter or olive oil spread and let it sit.

2. In your flat, wide bowl, begin to scramble your egg and add in the cinnamon.

3. One slice at a time, place your bread in the egg bowl, and make sure to coat the bread slices completely with the mixture. Give the bread time to soak up the egg fully, so after you have finished dipping both slices, there should be no egg mixture left in the bowl.

4. Now, place the soaked bread in your frying pan, and cook each side of each slice for about 2–3 minutes until you achieve a golden-brown hue.

5. To serve, the French toast, lay the bread on a medium plate while still hot, and top it with sliced bananas and pecan bits (or the toasted sunflower or pumpkin seeds) and drizzle some pure maple syrup over the top. Enjoy!

Tofu Breakfast Scramble

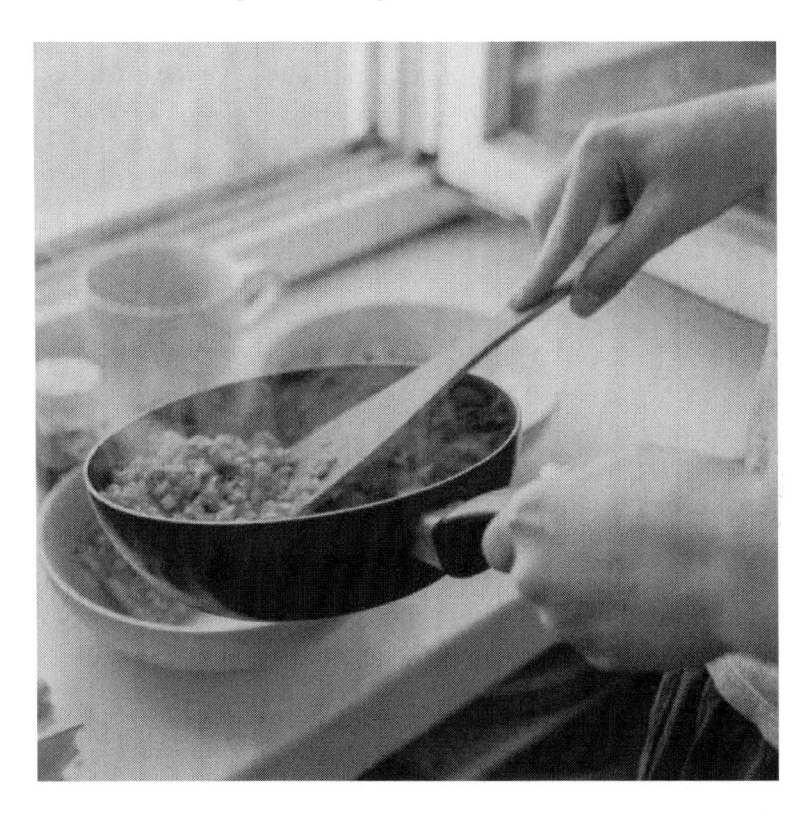

Vegan and vegetarian diets can be tricky to combine with the low-FODMAP diet. However, this breakfast recipe does it all and helps you have a nutritious, protein-rich meal in the morning to start your day! The plain tofu used in this recipe is a great alternative to other vegan proteins like lentils and beans, which are only low-FODMAP in low quantities. This savory breakfast is easy to change, depending on what you are craving for the day. It will keep you full for hours, especially if you pair this scramble with a slice of low-FODMAP bread. The tofu breakfast scramble takes under 10 minutes to cook and yields 1 full serving.

What You Will Need:
- 1 small to a medium mixing bowl
- 1 small to a medium frying pan
- 100 g of medium-firm or firm tofu
- ½ cup of grated carrots
- ½ cup of grated zucchini
- 1 tsp of soy sauce
- ¼ tsp of ground turmeric
- 2 tsp of cooking spray (or cooking oil)

Low-FODMAP Shopping Tips:
- Choose firm tofu so that you can be sure it is low-FODMAP. Although the ingredients list above suggests 100 g of firm tofu for the entire recipe, you can add more protein to your meal by using up to 160 g of tofu per serving.
- If you want to be extra cautious, you can swap normal soy sauce for its gluten-free version to make sure it is low-FODMAP.
- If you decide to pair this scramble with something, choose a low-FODMAP bread that contains no chickpea/garbanzo flour, coconut flour, soy flour, amaranth flour, or lupin flour. Also, try to avoid ingredients like concentrated fruit juices, pear juice, apple juice, inulin, apple fiber, high-fructose corn syrup, or honey. Wheat sourdough bread can be a good low-FODMAP option.

Method:
1. Begin by adding about ¼ cup of water to your mixing bowl. Stir in the soy sauce and ground

turmeric, and make sure to mix both well with the water.

2. Take your tofu and use your fingers to crumble it up, piece by piece. Let the bits fall into the mixing bowl and mix them with the water, soy sauce, and ground turmeric. Add in your grated or diced (based on personal preference) carrots and zucchini.

3. Add the cooking oil to your medium frying pan, and set it over a medium flame. Adding oil to this recipe helps give your tofu a yellowish color and will make the scramble look more like scrambled eggs.

4. Once the oil has begun to heat up, add the entire contents of the mixing bowl into the frying pan, and let everything cook through. You will know the tofu is ready when it has a sort of yellow or golden-brown color on all surfaces.

5. Serve the scramble on a plate with a slice of low-FODMAP bread and enjoy!

Although personalized methods are not made explicit in this recipe, do feel free to change your tofu scramble by adding in different spices and veggies or by topping your scramble with some type of garnish. You can also swap out the low-FODMAP bread with some low-FODMAP rice. Please make sure that you use this freedom responsibly! Check that everything you buy and the quantities you use for this recipe are all low-FODMAP. Enjoy your customizable tofu scramble!

Chapter 5: Lunch and Dinner Recipes

Rice-Based Recipes

Salmon Fried Rice

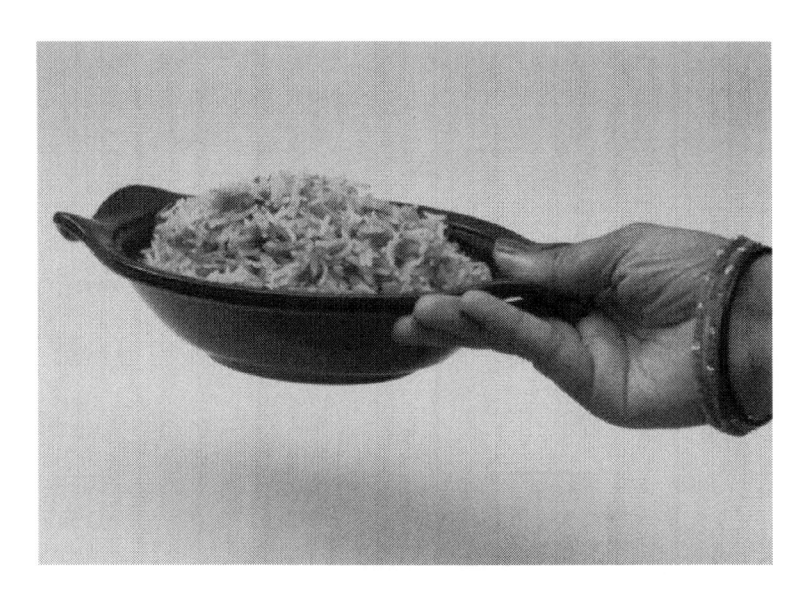

Many people on the low-FODMAP diet are looking for good sources of calcium since reintroducing dairy into your diet can take some easing into. Tinned salmon in this flavorful dish is an excellent source of protein that stays within the low-FODMAP diet guidelines! This particular recipe yields 3 servings and takes a total of 20 minutes, including preparation and cooking time.

What You Will Need:
- 1 large frying pan
- 1 medium saucepan

- 2 large eggs
- 1 large, peeled, and grated carrot
- 80 grams of green beans
- 1 sliced red bell pepper - deseeded
- ½ cup of finely chopped green onions/scallions (only use green part)
- 2 tbsp of ginger (crushed or grated fresh)
- 210 grams of canned plain pink salmon
- 1 cup uncooked rice (basmati or long-grain white rice)
  - OR use 2 cups precooked rice - this option will decrease total cook time
- 1 tbsp of garlic-infused oil
- 1 tbsp of sesame oil
- 2 tbsp of Nam Pla (Thai fish sauce)
- 2 tbsp of soy sauce
- Salt and Pepper

Low-FODMAP Shopping Tips:
- Buy garlic-infused oil that is free of garlic bits. We want to capture the garlic flavor without adding in the high-FODMAP fructans from the garlic itself
- If you want to be extra cautious, you can swap normal soy sauce for its gluten-free version to make sure it is low-FODMAP.
- Make sure the canned salmon you buy is plain and contains no onions or garlic. An alternative to canned salmon is to buy fresh and cook it before integrating it into this recipe.
- If you buy crushed ginger, make sure it is only ginger and that it contains no garlic.

Method:

1. Begin cooking rice in the saucepan according to packet instructions. Move on to step 2 if you are using precooked rice.

2. Prepare the vegetables as you would like. Suggestions have been included in the ingredient list above.

3. Heat the large frying pan over medium heat and add the garlic-infused oil and sesame oil. Add in the garlic and scallions and cook for not more than 2 minutes until translucent and you can smell the aroma of garlic. Add the slices of bell pepper and sauté for a full minute until softened. Then add green beans, tinned salmon (should be drained from a can), and carrot and stir until salmon breaks into bite-size pieces. At this point, turn the heat down slightly and add in the Thai fish sauce. Crack the eggs into the pan and continually stir all ingredients together until the eggs are fully cooked.

4. Add freshly cooked rice to the frying pan and stir in the soy sauce. Season with salt and pepper if desired.

5. Remove from heat once the dish is thoroughly and evenly heated. Plate and enjoy!

Japanese Rice/Sushi Balls

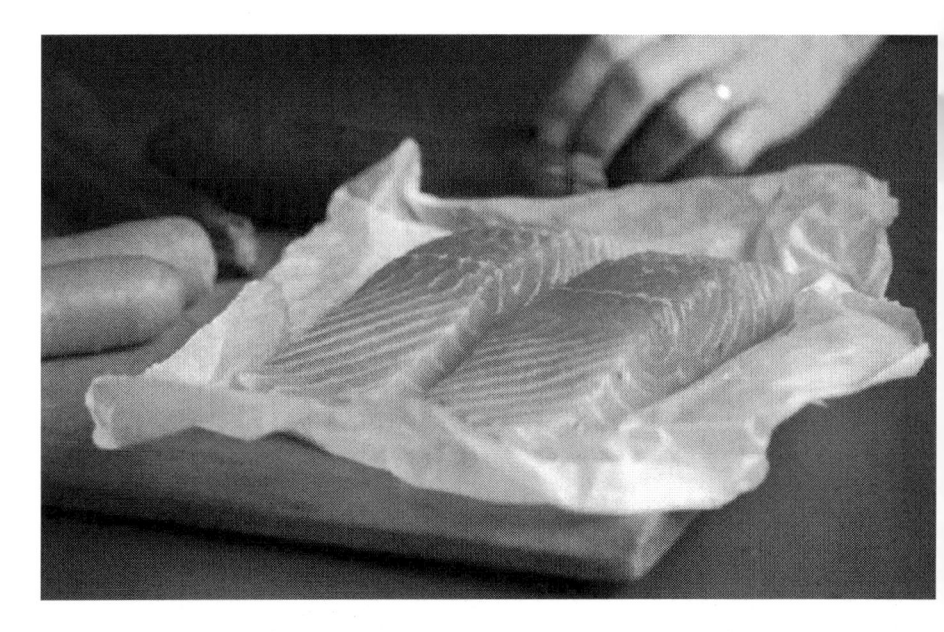

This low-calorie recipe is perfect for people who are on the go! The recipe serves 4 and only takes 20 minutes to prepare.

What You Will Need:
- 1 large mixing bowl
- 4 cups of baby spinach
- 1 small cucumber
- 1 large carrot
- 2 oranges
- 210 g of canned plain pink salmon
- 250 g of microwave quick-cook medium-grain brown rice (uncooked)
- 1 nori sheet (seaweed sheet)
- 3 tbsp of rice wine vinegar
- 3 tbsp of sesame seeds

- ¼ cup of mayonnaise
- 1 tbsp of sunflower, canola, OR rice bran oil (natural oil)
- 2 and ½ tbsp of low-FODMAP sweet chili sauce
- 1 tsp of soy sauce

Low-FODMAP Shopping Tips:
- Make sure the canned salmon you buy is plain and contains no onions or garlic. An alternative to canned salmon is to buy fresh and cook it before integrating it into this recipe.
- Choose a sweet chili sauce that contains no honey, high-fructose syrup, onion, or garlic. If that is difficult to find, you can always create the sauce from scratch using our low-FODMAP recipe that will be listed as an extra below this recipe.
- Nori (seaweed) sheets should be stocked in normal supermarkets but will be abundant in your local Asian market.
- Choose a mayonnaise that contains no garlic or onion.
- If you want to be extra cautious, you can swap normal soy sauce for its gluten-free version to make sure it is low in FODMAP.

Method:
1. Cook your rice in the microwave as per the packet instructions. Pour 2 tbsp of rice wine vinegar into the rice and set aside to let it soak.

2. Drain the canned salmon and crush the seaweed sheet into smaller flakes. Combine the rice,

mayonnaise, shredded nori, and salmon in a large bowl and mix the ingredients well.

3. Use wet hands to roll the mixture into small balls, tablespoon by tablespoon. Keeping your palms and fingers wet will help you avoid getting rice stuck in your hands. Roll and lightly cover each sushi ball in sesame seeds.

4. Combine the remaining rice wine vinegar, sweet chili sauce, natural oil, and soy sauce in a small bowl until they are well-mixed.

5. Peel the cucumber, carrot, and oranges and then appropriately dice or ribbon the vegetables. Combine with spinach into your serving bowl.

6. Plate the sushi balls by placing them over the salad you just prepared. Don't forget to drizzle some of the sweet chili sauce dressing. Enjoy!

Add-On: Low-FODMAP Sweet Chili Sauce

A low-FODMAP chili sauce can be difficult to find because most of them contain garlic. This is a fun recipe that follows the guidelines of a low-FODMAP diet and still gives you all the flavors of a store-bought sweet chili sauce! This recipe takes about 15 minutes to prepare, 30 minutes to cook, and yields about 500 mL of the sauce.

What You Will Need:
- 1 medium saucepan
- Preserving jar or container

- 1 food processor
- 1 and ½ cup of white vinegar
- 150 g of red chili (mild)
- 1 and ½ cup of white sugar

Method:
1. Wash your preserving jar with hot, soapy water, and place the jar in the oven at 250°F for 20 minutes so the jar can air dry and sterilize.

2. Roughly chop 50 g of the red chilies as they are and deseed. Roughly chop the remaining 200 g of the chilies. Add the chilies to the food processor with ½ cup of white vinegar and process them until they are very finely chopped.

3. Place a saucepan on the stove, heating it on low flame. When warm enough, pour the prepared chili mixture into the pan. Add in the white sugar and the remaining white vinegar, and stir it occasionally for about 5 minutes. The sugar should dissolve completely.

4. Wait for the mixture to boil and then simmer, occasionally stirring the sauce for 20–25 minutes until it thickens. The thickening process will continue as the sauce cools.

5. Pour your finished sauce into the sterilized, airtight preserving jar and store it in the fridge for up to 3 months.

Pasta-Based Recipes

Baked Chicken Alfredo Pasta

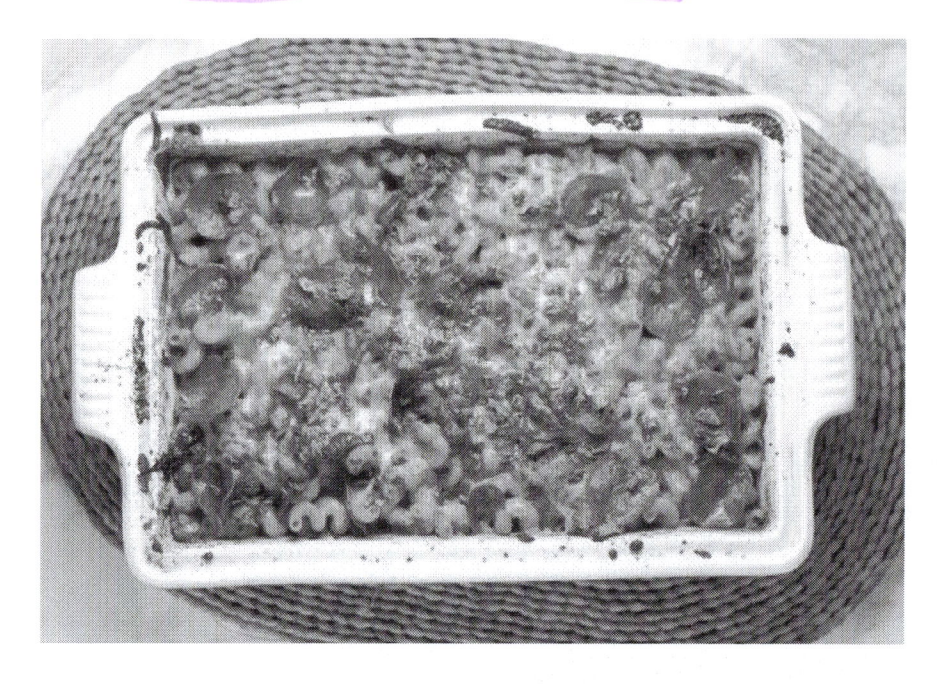

Here is your perfect comfort food lunch recipe! This one is really easy to adapt to your tastes and dietary restrictions. This meal also reheats well, and the leftovers are perfect for lunch the next day. Although this meal can take about 35 minutes of preparation time, the cooking happens in about 15 minutes, and you have 4 large servings of a wholesome meal!

What You Will Need:
- 1 large and 1 medium saucepan
- 1 large deep oven dish
- 1 large frying pan
- Olive oil, salt, pepper

- 450 g of chicken breast fillet
- 240 g of uncooked pasta (gluten-free)
- 2 cups of broccoli
- 4 cups of baby spinach
- ½ cup of green onions/scallions (only use the green part)
- 2 tbsp of fresh sage
- ½ tsp of dried basil
- ½ cup of a low-FODMAP cheese (optional: vegan cheese)
- 4 tbsp of olive oil (optional: dairy-free butter)
- 3 cups of a low-FODMAP milk
- ¼ cup of flour - gluten-free

Low-FODMAP Shopping Tips:
- If you buy vegan, soy-based cheese, ensure that it does not contain coconut flour onion or garlic.
- Choose a pure gluten-free pasta to avoid high-FODMAP ingredients like wheat, soy flour, amaranth flour, lupin flour, or inulin.
- Broccoli is low in FODMAP only in small servings, so try not to exceed the suggested serving size listed above.
- Choose a pure gluten-free flour that contains no chickpea/garbanzo flour, coconut flour, soy flour, amaranth flour, or lupin flour.
- Low-FODMAP cheeses include cheddar, parmesan, mozzarella, and Colby cheese.

Method:
1. Grease your deep oven dish and set your oven to preheat to 355°F. Begin boiling water in a large saucepan to cook your pasta

2. Chop your spinach, the green tips of your scallions, and the broccoli. Also, chop the chicken breast into smaller bite-size chunks.

3. In a large pan using a medium-to-high flame, heat olive oil until warm enough. Add the chicken and cook. When the hue of each side turns golden brown, remove it from the heat and set it to the side. Take advantage of the hot pan and cook the spinach until it begins to wilt. Place spinach on the side as well.

4. While the chicken is cooking, melt your dairy-free butter or heat some olive oil in another pan over a medium flame. When ready, add gluten-free flour, whisking together so that it creates a mixture. Continue stirring for 1 minute until the mixture becomes slightly frothy and then whisk in your low-FODMAP milk, ½ cup at a time. Season the mixture with basil, parmesan cheese (if you choose to use this), salt, and pepper. Grate your low-FODMAP cheese, and add half of it to the mixture in this frying pan. Stir only occasionally so that the mixture can thicken.

5. The water in your large saucepan should be boiling now. Add in your gluten-free pasta and cook for 5 minutes. Then, drain your pasta and toss with a little bit of olive oil.

6. Now, mix your broccoli, wilted spinach, green onions, cooked chicken, Alfredo sauce, and

cooked pasta, and place them in your oven dish. Top the dish with the remaining half of your grated cheese.

7. Bake the dish uncovered for 10 minutes and then grill for 2–3 minutes using the oven grill until the top of the dish is golden-brown.

8. Plate, top with the finely-chopped fresh sage, and enjoy!

Spaghetti Bolognese

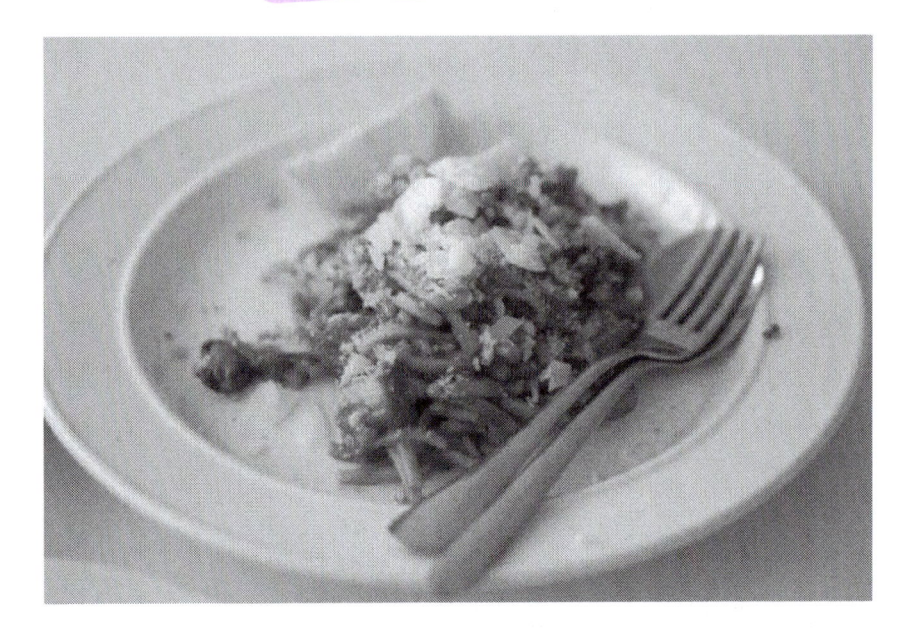

This comfort food is extremely easy to throw together and helps you bring the fresh flavors of Italy to your kitchen! The recipe will take you between 30–40 minutes to cook and will leave you with 4 full servings of spaghetti Bolognese!

What You Will Need:
- 1 large saucepan
- 1 large frying pan
- 1 medium saucepan
- 2 large carrots
- 160 g of green beans
- 1 tsp of dried basil
- 500 g of lean ground beef
- ½ cup of leeks (use only the green parts)
- ½ tsp of dried thyme

- 4 cups of baby spinach
- 400 g of canned crushed tomatoes
- Salt and pepper
- 2 tsp of olive oil
- 300 g of gluten-free spaghetti
- 1 tsp of dried oregano
- ½ cup of a low-FODMAP cheese (we recommend Colby or cheddar)
- 3 tbsp of tomato paste

<u>Low-FODMAP Shopping Tips:</u>
- Low-FODMAP cheeses include cheddar, parmesan, mozzarella, and Colby cheese. You can also choose to use vegan, soy-based cheese, but ensure that it does not contain coconut flour, onion, or garlic.
- Choose a pure gluten-free pasta to avoid high-FODMAP ingredients, like wheat, soy flour, amaranth flour, lupin flour, or inulin.
- The green tips of the leek are the low-FODMAP part, so buy leeks with long green stems.
- Choose a can of pure, crushed, or diced tomatoes to avoid potentially high-FODMAP ingredients like onion, garlic, or other spices/herbs. Also, make sure not to exceed the specified serving size for the canned tomatoes and tomato paste.

<u>Method:</u>
1. Begin by preparing your vegetables. Finely chop the green leek tips, roughly chop the baby spinach, slice the green beans into small bite-sized pieces, and peel and chop the carrots into long sticks.

2. Place the chopped veggies to the side, and place a big pan on the stove with medium flame. Warm the olive oil in the pan, and then add in your lean ground beef. Cook the meat until it has browned.

3. After the meat has cooked for a little while, begin to add in the tomato paste, canned tomatoes, chopped spinach and leek tips, oregano, thyme, and basil to the browned beef in the pan. Mix all of these ingredients, and allow the sauce to come to a mild boil in the pan. Bring the heat to low, and wait for the sauce to simmer. Make sure to stir often so the sauce doesn't burn or stick to the bottom of the pan. After 20 minutes, add some salt and pepper, to taste.

4. As the sauce is simmering, and you are stirring it every couple of minutes, boil the water in a big pot, add some salt to the water. When warm enough, add your gluten-free spaghetti, and cook it according to directions, and maintaining its al dente texture.

5. As the pasta boils, fill your medium saucepan with a little water, and place it on the stove to boil. Add the carrots and green beans to the boiling water, and let them cook and soften for not more than 3 minutes. After this, collect the veggies, transfer them to another plate, and set them to the side. You can either mince these cooked veggies in with the Bolognese sauce or serve separately on the side of your main meal.

6. Take the fully cooked spaghetti, draining the water, and pouring some olive oil. Toss the spaghetti, making sure the noodle is coated well. Finish cooking the bolognese sauce and remove it from the pan.

7. Serve the spaghetti in a large bowl, top it with Bolognese sauce, and then add in a sprinkle of your choice of low-FODMAP cheese. If you chose to keep the carrots and green beans separate, serve them on the side of your spaghetti Bolognese and enjoy!

Soups and Stews:

Lamb Stew

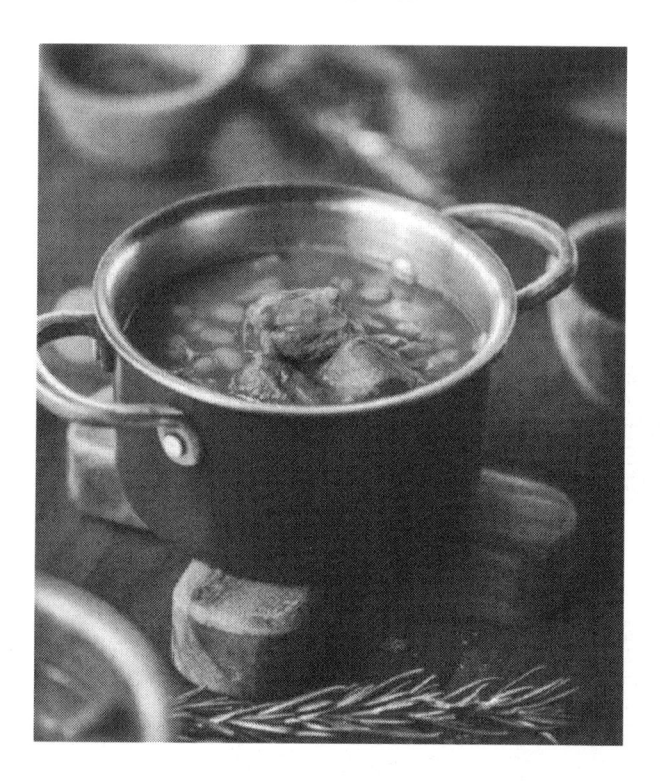

This simple stew is the perfect, easy-to-make winter comfort food. This meal is slow-cooked in 10 hours but only requires 20 minutes of preparation work from you. Try to get your ingredients in the slow cooker the night before if you're looking to have some stew for lunch and the morning if you're planning dinner. This recipe yields 4 full servings of stew.

What You Will Need:
- 1 slow cooker
- 1 medium frying pan

- 2 saucepans
- 500 g of lamb leg steaks
- 2 large carrots
- 180 g of green beans
- Salt and pepper
- 240 g of Japanese pumpkin (OR sweet potato or buttercup squash)
- 300 g of potato
- 8 slices of a low-FODMAP bread
- ½ tsp of dried thyme
- 1 tbsp of rice bran, sunflower, OR canola oil (natural oils)
- 1 tbsp of garlic-infused oil
- 1 and ½ cup of leeks (only use the green tips)
- 1 tsp of dried oregano
- 4 cups of a low-FODMAP chicken or beef stock
- 1 cup of boiling water
- 3 tbsp of fresh parsley

Low-FODMAP Shopping Tips:
- Buy garlic-infused oil that is free of garlic bits. We want to capture the garlic flavor without adding in the high-FODMAP fructans from the garlic itself
- The green tips of the leek are the low-FODMAP part, so buy leeks with long green stems.
- Buy low-FODMAP bread that contains no chickpea/garbanzo flour, coconut flour, soy flour, amaranth flour, or lupin flour. Also try to avoid ingredients like concentrated fruit juices, pear juice, apple juice, inulin, apple fiber, high-fructose corn syrup, or honey. Wheat sourdough bread can be a good low-FODMAP option.

- Choose a beef or chicken stock that does not contain any garlic or onion.

Method:
1. Grease the slow cooker and turn it on low. Begin boiling 1 cup of water, and mildly heat the beef or chicken stock in your saucepans.

2. Cut the lamb into cubes, making sure to remove the fat first. Brown the lamb for 4–5 minutes under medium flame. Once golden brown, add the lamb into the slow cooker.

3. Peel and chop the carrots, potato, and pumpkin into cubes. Roughly chop the green tips of the leeks. Pour the heated low-FODMAP stock, garlic-infused oil, thyme, and dried oregano into the slow cooker. Add in the veggies and pour over the boiling water. Season with salt and pepper.

4. Leave the stew in the slow cooker to cook for a minimum of 8 hours. Use low flame

5. When the cooking time is almost done, check the stew. If the meat is tender, mash up the stew to help it thicken. If the stew is a little dry, add enough boiling water to cover the ingredients and then mash.

6. Begin boiling water in a saucepan. Trim the green beans into small, bite-sized pieces and put them in the saucepan, cooking for 2–3 minutes. Place the

drained beans in the saucepan, stirring them into the stew.

7. Toast your bread, and chop up the fresh parsley.

8. Serve the stew with parsley garnish and bread on the side. Enjoy!

Salads

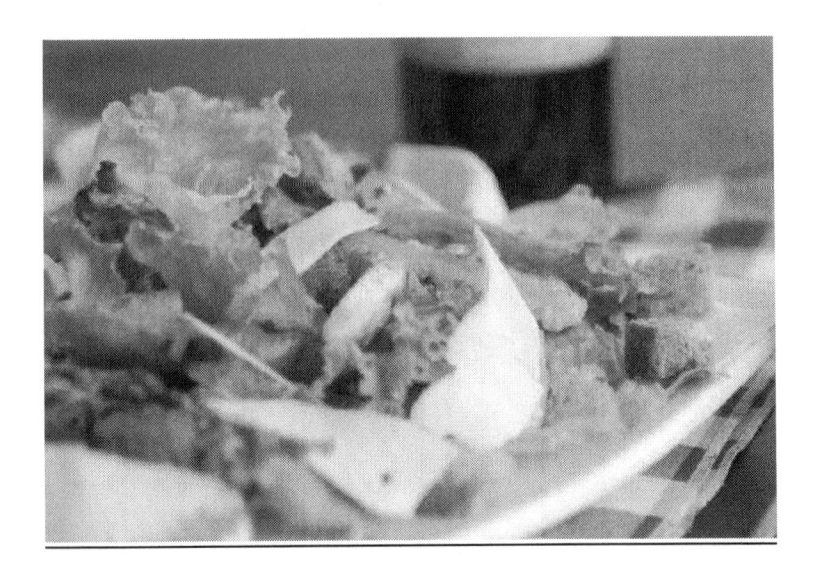

Moroccan-Inspired Chicken Salad with an Orange Dressing

This salad is not only nutritious and delicious but is also super quick and easy to toss together. Since there is no need to prepare the leftovers before eating them, this is the perfect meal to take to work, school, or anywhere on the go! In only 5 minutes of preparation time and 10 minutes of cook time, you are free to enjoy 2 servings of this Moroccan-spiced salad!

What You Will Need:
- 1 medium frying pan
- 2 Imperial mandarin oranges
- 1 tbsp of orange juice (freshly squeezed is preferred)
- ¼ tsp of ground cumin
- 2 cups of lettuce (assorted leaves are ok)

- 1 small cucumber
- 1 red bell pepper
- ⅛ tsp of ground ginger
- ½ tbsp of red wine vinegar
- 250 g of skinless chicken breast
- Salt and pepper
- ½ tsp of paprika
- ⅛ tsp of ground turmeric
- ¼ tsp of ground coriander
- ½ tbsp of garlic-infused oil
- ⅛ tsp of white sugar
- 2 tbsp of olive oil
- ½ tbsp of maple syrup - pure

Low-FODMAP Shopping Tips:
- Choose a pure maple syrup rather than maple-flavored syrup because that could contain high-FODMAP ingredients.
- Buy garlic-infused oil that is free of garlic bits. We want to capture the garlic flavor without adding in the high-FODMAP fructans from the garlic itself.
- Try and use fresh oranges to squeeze the orange juice and use for zest.

Method:
1. Mix the garlic-infused oil, turmeric, coriander, ground ginger, paprika, white sugar, and cumin in a bowl. Chop up the chicken into cubes, coat the pieces in the spice mixture, and dust with some pepper ground, and salt according to your preference.

2. Add the prepared chicken pieces to a frying pan over medium-to-high heat. Cook the chicken through until it is golden-brown on the outside, and then set it aside to cool.
   - It is best to make this salad with chicken that has completely cooled so that the heat from the meat doesn't cause the vegetables to wilt. You can even place the cooked chicken in the fridge.

3. Squeeze fresh orange juice and mix it in with red wine vinegar, pure maple syrup, olive oil, salt, and black pepper.

4. Deseed and dice the red bell pepper, peel and slice the cucumber, and peel and separate the slices of the mandarin oranges.

5. Assemble the ingredients in a salad bowl by placing the salad first and then topping with the chicken. Drizzle your homemade orange dressing over the cooled chicken and salad and enjoy!

Other Recipes

Mini Savory Crepes

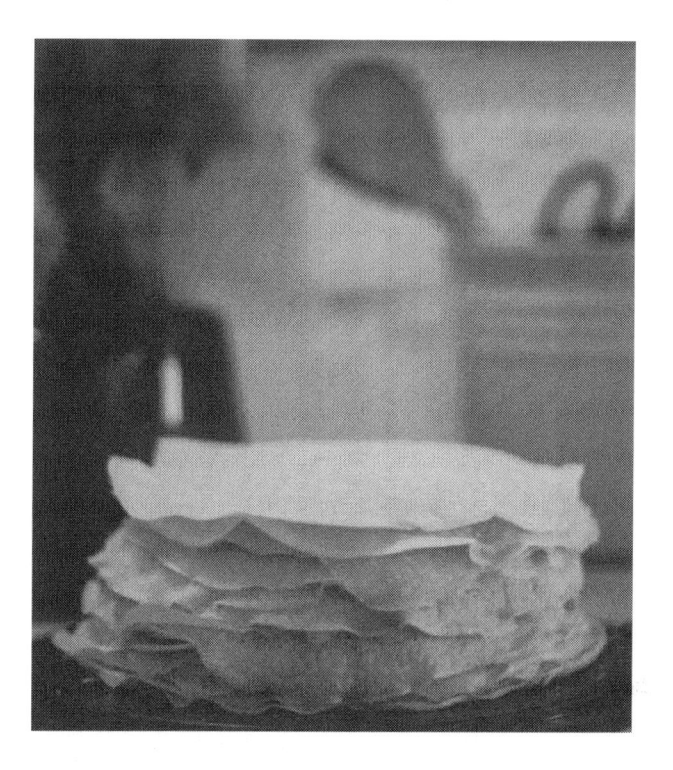

These mini crepes with a savory mince and mustard sauce are a great new low-FODMAP brunch idea for you! The different components of this meal store well, so this is the perfect meal-prep option! You can store the crepe preparations in the fridge for around four days, and cook everything just when you need it. The savory mince and mustard sauce also reheats well, so it won't feel as if you are eating leftovers. The recipe should take no more than a total of 35 minutes of cook time and will yield 4 servings of 2 mini crepes.

What You Will Need:

Crepe Batter
- 1 mixing bowl, large
- 1 frying pan, large
- 1 frying pan, medium
- 2 cups of low-FODMAP milk
- 1 saucepan, small
- 2 large eggs
- 1 mixing bowl, small
- 2 tbsp of olive oil spread (or dairy-free butter)
- 1 cup of gluten-free all-purpose flour
- ¼ tsp salt

Savory Mince
- ½ cup leeks (green parts only)
- 1 tsp of dried oregano
- 500 g of lean ground beef
- 4 cups of baby spinach
- ½ tbsp Worcestershire sauce
- 2 large carrots
- 1 tsp of dried basil
- 400 g of plain canned tomatoes (canned or diced)
- ½ tsp of dried thyme
- Salt and pepper

Mustard Sauce
- 1 large egg
- 1 cup of low-FODMAP chicken stock
- 2 tbsp white sugar
- ¼ cup of white vinegar
- 1 handful of fresh basil leaves
- 1 tbsp of gluten-free all-purpose flour

- 1 tsp yellow mustard powder

Low-FODMAP Shopping Tips:
- The green tips of the leek are the low-FODMAP part, so buy leeks with long green stems.
- Choose a pure gluten-free flour that contains no chickpea/garbanzo flour, coconut flour, soy flour, amaranth flour, or lupin flour.
- Choose a can of pure crushed or diced tomatoes to avoid potentially high-FODMAP ingredients like onion, garlic, or other spices/herbs. Also, make sure not to exceed the specified serving size for the canned tomatoes.
- Choose a chicken stock that does not contain any garlic or onion.
- Most store-bought Worcestershire sauces are low-FODMAP in the suggested serving size listed above because although they do contain small amounts of onion and garlic, they are fermented in the production process which helps reduce the FODMAP levels in the sauce.

Method:
1. Begin by melting the dairy-free olive oil spread or dairy-free butter you have chosen into a large mixing bowl. Add in your low-FODMAP milk, gluten-free all-purpose flour, and salt into the bowl and mix everything. In a small mixing bowl, whisk your eggs together, and add them into the larger mixing bowl. Stir or whisk this mixture together until it is completely smooth and homogenous. Set aside the batter until you get to step 5.

2. Now, begin to prepare your veggies. Finely chop the spinach and green tops from the leeks, and peel and grate the carrots.

3. Begin to prepare the mustard sauce next by placing a small saucepan on very low heat. In the pot, whisk the egg together with the white sugar and then add the mustard powder, white vinegar, gluten-free all-purpose flour, and chicken stock to the pot. Keep lightly heating this sauce throughout the rest of the cooking process and let the sauce thicken. Stir occasionally to avoid burning it.

4. Now, begin cooking the savory mince. Heat a big frying pan using medium-to-high flame over the stove, and add in a splash of olive oil or some other low-FODMAP cooking oil. Place the ground beef in the pan, and add the finely chopped green leek leaves. Lightly fry the lean ground beef until it begins to brown, making sure to stir it every so often. Then, add half your spinach and carrots to the pan, followed by your canned, diced, or crushed tomatoes. Add as well the dried oregano, dried thyme, dried basil, Worcestershire sauce, and salt and pepper, to taste. Mix everything in the pan together well and let it come to a light boil. Reduce the heat to low or medium, and let the sauce simmer until you are done cooking the crepes. Stir occasionally to avoid burning it.

5. While the beef mince is simmering, place your medium frying pan over medium-high heat, and

spray the entire base of the pan with low-FODMAP cooking oil. Using a measuring cup (or you can just "eyeball it"), scoop out about 1/4 cup of the crepe batter you had set aside earlier, and pour it into the frying pan. Lift the pan with the handle and tilt the pan in each direction so that the batter covers the entire base of the pan in an even layer. Cook the crepe until the bottom side is a light golden brown, which should take about 2 minutes, and then flip the crepe over. Finish cooking the top side of the crepe, and remove from the heat, and set aside. Repeat this process until you have used up all of the batters, which should yield about 8 crepes. You can store the cooked crepes inside the oven (keep the oven off) to keep them warm and fresh until you serve them.

6. At this point, check to see if your mustard sauce has thickened and if your beef mince is heated evenly. Remove everything from the heat and prepare to serve.

7. Serve the mince and the other half of the chopped baby spinach and carrots inside the crepes (you can roll or fold up the crepes), and then drizzle the mustard sauce over the finished dish. Top the crepes with a handful of basil leaves if you'd like to and enjoy!

Lamb Kebabs

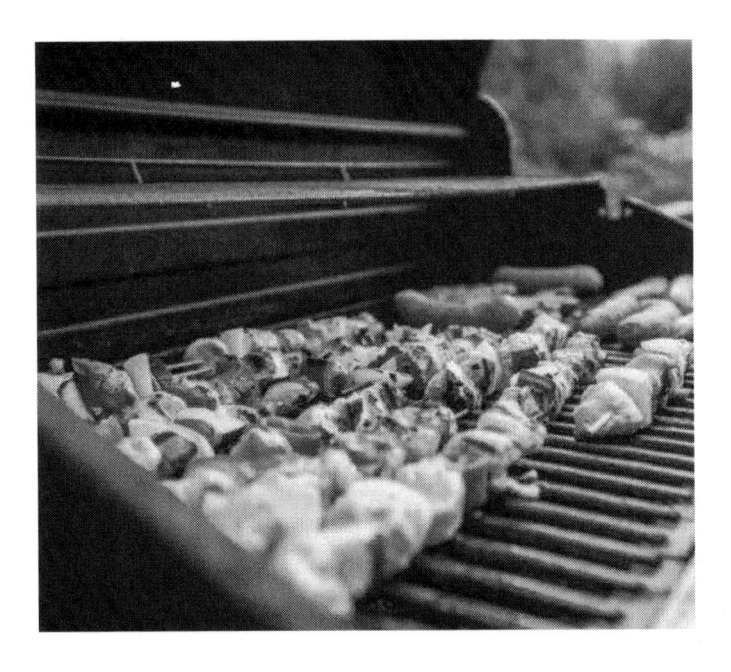

These juicy BBQ lamb skewers are served with a drizzle of lemon yogurt dressing and a side of mashed potatoes—delicious! The flavors in this meal will make you forget that you are following a low-FODMAP diet and will help you in your elimination phase and beyond. This recipe is also extremely customizable and will also help you clear extra or older veggies out of your fridge. The method will show you how to cook these skewers in a frying pan on the stove, but you can also cook using a BBQ if you have one. This meal should take you about 30 minutes to make once you have marinated the lamb for a few hours or overnight, and it will leave you with 4 servings!

What You Will Need:

Lamb Skewers
- 1 shallow dish
- 3 tbsp of lemon juice
- 1 large frying pan
- 1 pack of wooden skewers
- 1 tsp of dried oregano
- 600 g of lamb steak legs
- 200 g of zucchini
- 2 tbsp of fresh parsley
- 1 red bell pepper
- 3 tbsp of garlic-infused oil
- ¼ tsp of dried thyme
- Salt and pepper

Slaw
- 1 mixing bowl
- 2 cups of red cabbage
- 2 cups of iceberg lettuce
- ¼ cup of green onions/scallions (only use green part)

Mashed Potatoes
- 1 large saucepan
- 1 potato masher
- 800 g of potato
- Salt
- 1 pinch of dried oregano
- 2 tsp of olive oil

Yogurt Dressing
- 1 small mixing bowl
- 2 tbsp of lemon juice
- ½ cup of lactose-free or coconut yogurt

- 1 and ½ tbsp of fresh parsley
- ¼ tsp garlic-infused oil

Low-FODMAP Shopping Tips:
- Buy garlic-infused oil that is free of garlic bits. We want to capture the garlic flavor without adding in the high-FODMAP fructans from the garlic itself.
- Try to use fresh lemon juice for this recipe.
- Savoy cabbage can be high in FODMAP so when buying ingredients for the slaw, make sure to choose low-FODMAP red/purple cabbage or go with regular cabbage.
- Choose low-FODMAP yogurt that is free of inulin, lactose, agave syrup, fruit juice, honey, fructose, high-fructose corn syrup, and high-FODMAP fruits.

Method:
1. Begin by chopping all the lamb into small bite-sized chunks. In your shallow dish or bowl, add in and mix the garlic-infused oil, thyme, oregano, lemon juice, parsley, and black pepper to taste. Add the lamb chunks into this mixture, and marinate the meat in the fridge, preferably overnight, but a minimum of 4 hours would suffice.

2. Once the lamb has marinated at the desired time, bring it out of the fridge. Deseed your red bell pepper, and slice it into chunks. Thickly slice the zucchini as well. Now, begin making the kebabs by sliding the lamb, red bell pepper, and zucchini onto your skewers in a pattern. It is up to you how

full you want each skewer to be and how many veggies you would like to slide onto each one.

3. Now, begin to prepare your slaw by slicing or chopping up your red cabbage and iceberg lettuce. Finely chop the green chips of your green onions and toss them into a mixing bowl with the cabbage and lettuce.

4. Begin to prepare the potatoes by peeling them and roughly chopping them into smaller pieces. In a large saucepan, bring water to a boil and add in the potatoes. Let them cook until they are fully tender. This should take about 15–20 minutes and will take less time the smaller your potato chunks are.

5. As the potatoes are cooking, place a medium frying pan over medium heat. Add in a drizzle of cooking oil (make sure it is low-FODMAP cooking oil! You can alternatively use some more garlic-infused oil), and let it heat up in the pan. Place the lamb skewers in the pan and cook for about 2–3 minutes on each side until the meat is cooked to your liking. Once you have cooked the meat according to your preference, remove the skewers from the heat and set them aside to rest.

6. At this point, the potatoes should be tender and cooked. Drain them and drizzle them with olive oil, some salt, and oregano. Begin to mash the potatoes with a potato masher (you can also use a

fork or other utensil to mash) and make sure the oil and spices have mixed fully.

7. Lastly, we will prepare the lemon yogurt dressing. In a small mixing bowl, add in your choice of low-FODMAP yogurt, and mix it with garlic-infused oil, parsley, and lemon juice. You can add in a pinch of sugar if the flavor of this dressing is a little too sharp for your liking. Stir fast so that everything is well-mixed together, and there are no clumps in the dressing.

8. Place the lamb skewers on a large serving plate and drizzle with the dressing we just prepared. Serve with mashed potatoes on the side and enjoy!

Chicken Enchiladas

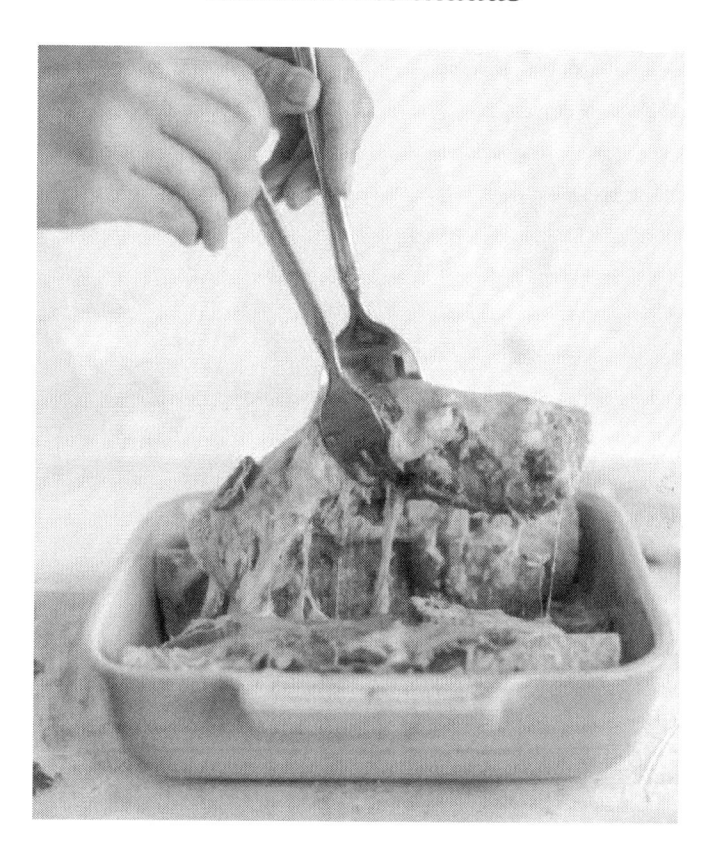

Mexican food can be hard to integrate into a low-FODMAP diet because it is largely based on gluten products, beans, garlic, and onions. However, this recipe manages to follow all low-FODMAP guidelines (even the most restrictive guidelines for the elimination phase) and still tastes extremely authentic. A lot of store-bought ingredients for this recipe would naturally be high-FODMAP choices, so we make the generally store-bought parts of this recipe from scratch. The enchiladas still will not take more than 15 minutes to prepare. Cooking time is less than an hour, most of which happens in the oven.

This recipe yields a full 6 servings of this delicious comfort food.

What You Will Need:

From-Scratch Enchilada Sauce
- 1 medium-sized saucepan
- ¼ cup garlic-infused oil (OR ¼ cup of onion infused oil)
- 415 g of diced tomatoes - canned
- ¼ cup of all-purpose flour (gluten-free)
- 2 tsp of red chili powder
- 2 cups of low-FODMAP chicken stock
- ½ tsp of salt
- ½ tsp of cumin
- ½ tsp of oregano

Actual Enchiladas
- 1 large mixing bowl
- 1 large nonstick skillet
- 1 small plate
- ½ tsp of oregano (can use more to taste)
- 1 small mixing bowl
- 1 oven-safe glass dish (13 x 19 inches, or something equivalent)
- Freshly ground black pepper
- 680 g of boneless, skinless chicken breast
- 1 cup of Havarti cheese
- 2 tsp of garlic-infused oil (OR 2 tsp of onion infused oil)
- ¼ cup of cilantro
- ½ cup of green onions/scallions (only use green part)

- ¼ tsp of red chili powder
- 10 corn tortillas
- 115 g of fresh green chilies
- 1 cup of sharp cheddar cheese (can use extra sharp cheddar cheese)
- 200 g of feta cheese
- ½ tsp of salt
- ½ tsp of cumin (can use more to taste)

Low-FODMAP Shopping Tips:
- The cheeses in their quantities listed just above are all low-FODMAP options, but if you decide to choose vegan cheeses, check to make sure what you buy contains no garlic or onion.
- Choose a pure gluten-free all-purpose flour that contains no chickpea/garbanzo flour, coconut flour, soy flour, lentil flour, amaranth flour, or lupin flour.
- Buy garlic-infused oil that is free of garlic bits. We want to capture the garlic flavor without adding in the high-FODMAP fructans from the garlic itself. The same guideline stands if you choose to use onion-infused oil.
- Choose a chicken stock that does not contain any garlic or onion.

Method:
1. First, we will begin by preparing the red enchilada sauce from scratch. Take your saucepan, and set it over a medium flame. Add in your oil and let it heat quite a bit in the pot. At this point, add in your flour a little at a time and whisk while it mixes in and cooks with the oil for about a minute

or two. This will help cook out the raw flour taste from the finished sauce.

2. Once that is lightly cooked, whisk in your chili powder and stir for about 30 seconds. Then, slowly begin to add the rest of the ingredients in the following order: chicken stock, canned diced tomatoes, cumin, salt, and oregano. Stir these ingredients together to mix well, and then let the mixture sit in the pot and come to a light boil. Let the sauce simmer and heat thoroughly for about 10 minutes and then remove from heat and set aside. This method will make about 3 cups of sauce. You are free to use this entire quantity for the enchiladas, but if you don't need it all, you can store it in the fridge in a covered container for up to 2 weeks.

3. As the sauce is simmering for those 10 minutes, you can begin preparing the enchiladas. Start by dicing the chicken into smaller pieces and place them into your large mixing bowl. Add the cumin, salt, oregano, chili powder, and black pepper to taste into the mixing bowl with the chicken. Toss the chicken chunks to coat them completely with all these spices.

4. Put your large non-stick skillet over a medium flame, and add the oil you have chosen for the enchiladas. Heat the oil and then add the coated chicken pieces into the pan. Let the chicken cook for about 3–5 minutes until it is just beginning to

lose its natural pink color or when it is halfway cooked.

5. At this point, the from-scratch red sauce should be ready to take off the heat. Add in a splash of this into the pan with the chicken, along with your minced green chilies, and fully coat the chicken in this. Continue cooking the chicken in the pan for another 3–5 minutes until it is completely cooked and heated all the way through.

6. Now, you can prepare the oven that has been preheated to 350 degrees Fahrenheit. Use a rack when cooking this dish in the oven, and place it in the middle of your oven. Coat the bottom of your baking dish with a little bit of your enchilada red sauce.

7. Now, place your shredded cheddar and Havarti cheeses into a small mixing bowl, and mix them evenly. On a small plate, set one corn tortilla down and coat its entire surface with the red sauce. Place a small amount of cooked chicken down the middle of the tortilla and lightly sprinkle some cheese from the small mixing bowl on top. Roll up the tortilla and place it, face down, into your oven dish. Repeat this process until you have used up all the corn tortillas, all the chicken, and about 1/3 of the shredded cheese mix. Again, you can choose how much red sauce to use for each step in this recipe. Place all the tortilla rolls close together in the oven dish.

8. Pour a good amount of the remaining enchilada sauce over the rolled tortillas in the oven dish and distribute the remaining cheese (about 2/3 of the starting amount) over the rolled tortillas. Evenly crumble the feta cheese over the top and bake for about 20–30 minutes. Remove the dish from the oven once the enchiladas have cooked and the cheese is golden brown and bubbly.

9. Finally, top the baked dish with your finely chopped scallions and cilantro, and divide the dish into 6 even servings. Eat one and share or save the rest. Enjoy!

Chapter 6: Tasty Snack Recipes

Lemon Zucchini Muffins

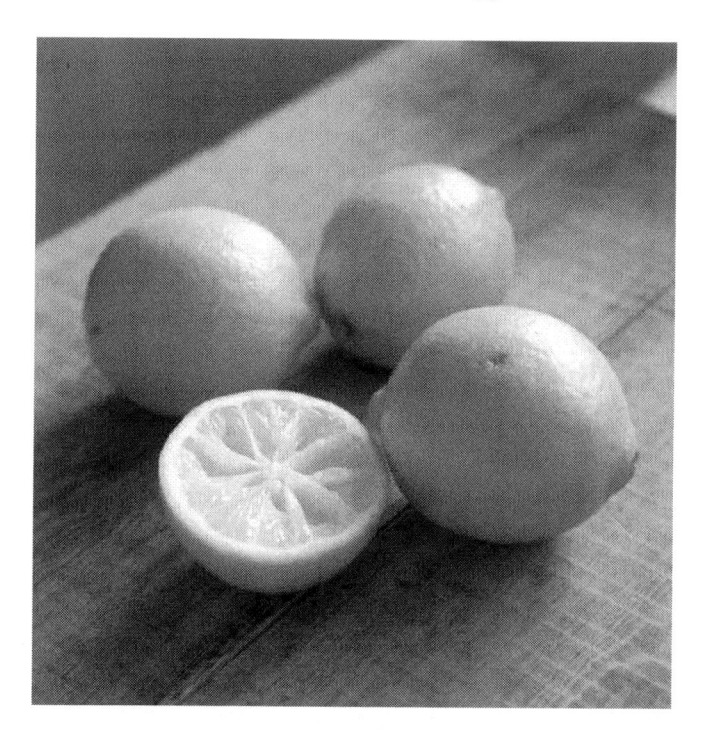

These perfectly fluffy and moist lemon poppyseed muffins are not only delicious, but they also have added health benefits from the zucchini! We have listed this recipe in the Snacks section, but these muffins also make a great breakfast for people on the go. Each ingredient adds a unique flavor that will take your taste buds to a whole new world, and you won't believe zucchini tastes so much like a baked good. The recipe only takes 10 minutes of preparation before baking and you will have 9 golden brown, wonderfully textured muffins at the end. The serving size is 1 muffin.

What You Will Need:
- 1 large mixing bowl
- 1 cup of gluten-free all-purpose flour
- 1 muffin tin (with at least 9 spots)
- 3 tsp of poppy seeds
- 180 g of zucchini
- ½ tsp of baking soda
- 1 large egg
- 1 tbsp of lemon juice
- 1 tsp baking powder
- 1 tbsp of lemon zest
- ¾ cup of tightly packed brown sugar
- 1 tsp of vanilla extract
- ½ cup of olive oil
- ½ tsp of salt

Low-FODMAP Shopping Tips
- Choose a pure, gluten-free flour that contains no chickpea/garbanzo flour, coconut flour, soy flour, lentil flour, amaranth flour, or lupin flour.
- Try to use fresh lemon juice and fresh lemon zest.

Method:
1. Begin by preheating your oven to 350° F, and grease nine of the spots in your muffin tin.

2. Grate your zucchini and then place everything on a clean tea towel. Wrap the tea towel around the grated zucchini and drain the excess water by squeezing the zucchini in the sink. This step is extremely important, and you should not skip it. Otherwise, your muffins will come out of the oven soggy from the zucchini's excess water.

3. Set the grated zucchini aside after step two, and move on the making the muffin batter. In your large mixing bowl, whisk together your egg, along with the brown sugar, lemon juice, lemon zest, olive oil, and vanilla extract. Once all your liquids are mixed, slowly mix the salt, baking soda, flour, and baking powder. Once these ingredients are all mixed, slowly fold in the grated zucchini and all the poppyseeds. Stir the batter until everything is evenly mixed.

4. Now, you can pour (or scoop using a ¼ cup measuring cup) batter into the nine spots you greased on the baking pan earlier. Make sure to split the batter as evenly as possible to avoid overfilling any spot.

5. Set the baking tin into the oven and bake for about 15 minutes. Before pulling the muffins out, put a toothpick or fork into the center of one or two muffins to make sure it comes out completely clean. Once you are sure the muffins are done cooking, pull them out from the oven, let them cool down, and enjoy!!

Garlic Bread

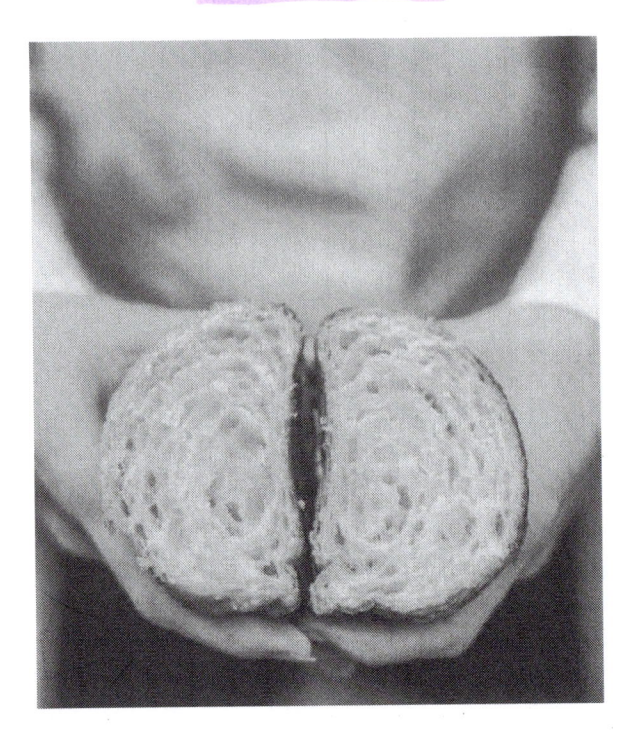

You might have said goodbye to garlic bread when you first picked up this diet's elimination phase, but here is a recipe for garlic bread that easily fits into the guidelines of the diet! This garlic bread is a perfect snacking material, but you can also use this to pair with some of your other low-FODMAP meal options. Although the recipe manages to be low in FODMAP, it is, by no means, healthy. It is downright delicious as well. For that reason, please be cautious, and make sure to stay true to the suggested serving size. This recipe only has 5 ingredients; it will take you only 15 minutes to complete, yielding 3 servings of 4 pieces each. Indulge!

What You Will Need:

- 1 small bowl
- 1 small baking tray
- 6 slices of a low-FODMAP bread
- 4 tbsp of olive oil spread or a dairy-free butter
- 1 pinch of oregano
- 1 pinch of salt
- 3 tbsp of garlic-infused oil

Low-FODMAP Shopping Tips:
- Buy garlic-infused oil that is free of garlic bits. We want to capture the garlic flavor without adding in the high-FODMAP fructans from the garlic itself.
- Buy low-FODMAP bread that contains no chickpea/garbanzo flour, coconut flour, soy flour, amaranth flour, or lupin flour. Also try to avoid ingredients like concentrated fruit juices, pear juice, apple juice, inulin, apple fiber, high-fructose corn syrup, or honey. Wheat sourdough bread can be a good low-FODMAP option.

Method:
1. Begin by slicing the bread into triangles and removing the crusts if you would like to.

2. In a small glass bowl, melt together your dairy-free spread with the garlic-infused oil and mix them well.

3. Prepare your oven tray by placing a baking sheet over the entire surface.

4. Now, take each triangle of the bread, and dip it into the butter mixture, making sure to coat the

entire piece of bread. Place each coated triangle of bread onto the baking tray, making sure to leave sufficient space between each piece.

5. Sprinkle the tops of the bread with salt and oregano and then place the baking tray into the oven for about 5 minutes. Once the tops are golden brown, flip the pieces over, sprinkle more oregano and salt, and continue baking for another 3-5 minutes.

6. Once both sides are done baking and the garlic bread has a golden-brown color on both sides, serve the pieces immediately. Enjoy!

Frozen Yogurt Bark

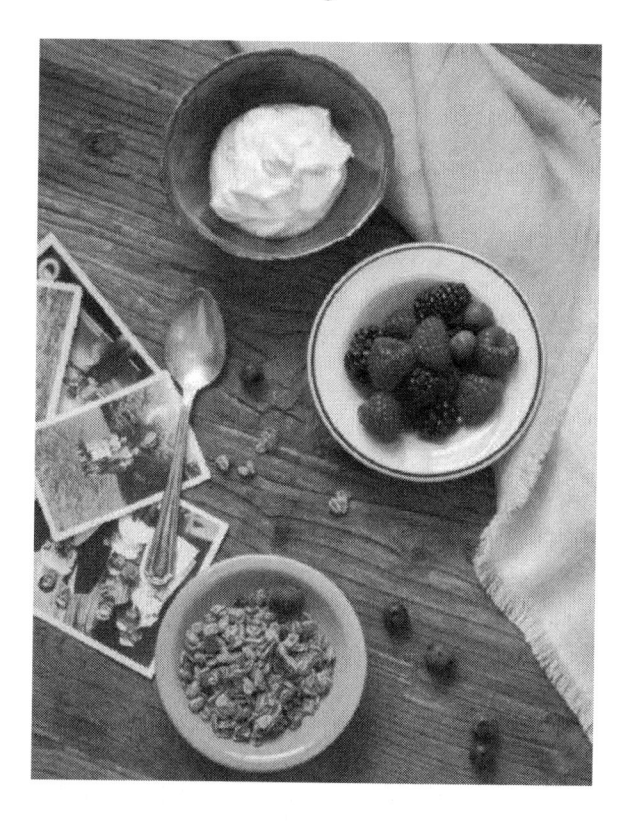

Sometimes, all we are craving is a frozen treat, and ice cream can be tough to integrate into a low-FODMAP diet. Instead of other frozen treats that could potentially flare your IBS symptoms, go ahead and try this frozen yogurt with berries! The freezing process will take about 3 hours, but the preparation itself takes only 5 minutes! You will be able to make 10 servings of this delicious snack in a very short amount of time.

What You Will Need:
- 1 large baking tray
- 1 mixing bowl

- 300 g of lactose-free yogurt (a coconut yogurt is also an option)
- 5 strawberries
- 15 blueberries
- 1 tsp vanilla extract
- 8 raspberries
- 2 tbsp strawberry jam

Low-FODMAP Shopping Tips:
- Choose low-FODMAP yogurt that is free of inulin, lactose, agave syrup, fruit juice, honey, fructose, high-fructose corn syrup, and high-FODMAP fruits.
- Choose a jam that does not contain the following high-FODMAP ingredients: fructose-glucose syrup, high fructose corn syrup, fruit juice concentrate, apple or pear juice, agave syrup, honey, inulin, or fructose. Instead, opt for a jam that is sweetened with low-FODMAP ingredients like glucose syrup, corn syrup, sucrose, or dextrose.

Method:
1. Cover the surface of your baking tray with baking or parchment paper.

2. In your mixing bowl, combine your yogurt and vanilla extract. Scoop the yogurt out into the prepared baking tray and flatten it out so that the yogurt is just under an inch thick. It should still be thick enough to hold the fruit that you will push in it.

3. Melt your jam in the microwave or a saucepan over the stove. Once it has thinned down, pour it into the center of the baking tray, and use a spoon to swirl the melted jam throughout the yogurt.

4. Chop your fresh strawberries into small bite-size pieces and sprinkle the chunks over the yogurt in the baking tray. Add in your blueberries and crumble the raspberries into the yogurt as well.

5. Place the entire baking tray into the freezer, and let it sit for at least 3 hours until it has hardened.

6. Pull the yogurt bark out after a few hours and use a sharp knife to cut the bark into about 10 pieces. You can eat them immediately and share them with friends, or you can place the bark in the freezer while wrapped in a vacuum container. Take them out whenever you want to have some. Enjoy!

Chicken Quinoa Meatballs

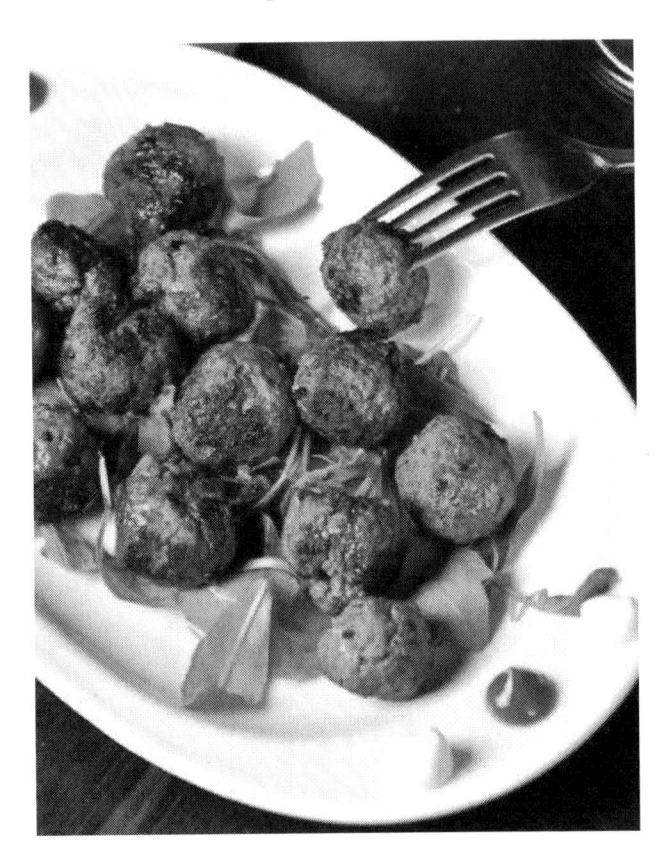

This recipe is perfect for making a quick snack, appetizer, or even a main meal if you serve with low-FODMAP rice. Since it is so versatile, we had to include the recipe in this book! This section also includes instructions that teach you how to make a teriyaki sauce from scratch that you can serve with the chicken quinoa meatballs. The snack will take you about 45 minutes to prepare and will yield 4 servings of about 5 meatballs each.

What You Will Need:

Chicken Quinoa Meatballs
- 1 mesh sieve
- 1 medium saucepan
- 1 large mixing bowl
- 1 large baking tray
- 1 small saucepan
- ¼ cup of quinoa
- 500 g of ground chicken
- 1 large egg
- 2 tbsp of gluten-free all-purpose flour (use as needed)
- 1 tsp brown sugar
- ⅔ cup of water
- 1 tsp of olive oil
- ½ cup of green onions/scallions (only use green part)
- ½ cup of fresh cilantro
- 1 tsp of crushed ginger
- 1 tbsp of lime juice
- ½ tsp of lime zest
- Salt and pepper
- 2 tsp of sesame seeds
- 2 tsp of Thai fish sauce (Nam Pla)
- ¼ tsp of dried red chili flakes

Teriyaki Sauce
- ½ cup of water
- 2 tsp of crushed ginger
- 2 tbsp of brown sugar
- 2 tsp of cornstarch
- 4 tbsp of soy sauce
- 1 and ½ tbsp of garlic-infused oil
- 2 tbsp of rice wine vinegar

- 1 tsp of sesame oil

Low-FODMAP Shopping Tips
- Choose cornstarch that is made from maize and not from wheat to ensure that it is low-FODMAP cornstarch.
- Choose a bottle of crushed ginger that does not contain garlic. It should be purely grated ginger. If you are concerned, you can opt to buy fresh ginger and grate it yourself.
- Ensure that your dried chili flakes do not contain any garlic or onion powder.
- If you want to be extra cautious, you can swap normal soy sauce for its gluten-free version to make sure it is low in FODMAP.
- Buy garlic-infused oil that is free of garlic bits. We want to capture the garlic flavor without adding in the high-FODMAP fructans from the garlic itself.
- Choose a pure gluten-free flour that contains no chickpea/garbanzo flour, coconut flour, soy flour, lentil flour, amaranth flour, or lupin flour.

Method:
1. Begin by preheating your oven to 400°F and lining your large baking tray with baking paper or greasing the tray.

2. Pour the quinoa into your mesh sieve, and rinse it thoroughly under cold water for 30–40 seconds. Rinsing will help remove the naturally bitter flavor from the quinoa. Then, drizzle olive oil into a medium saucepan and place the pot over medium to high heat. Add the quinoa, and let it

toast in the olive oil for about a minute before adding the water and bringing the contents of the pot to a boil. Turn the heat down slightly and allow the quinoa to simmer for about 12–15 minutes until it is cooked. You will know the quinoa is done cooking once all the water has evaporated and the rings have sprouted from the quinoa. Remove the quinoa from the heat and set it aside.

3. While the quinoa cooks, prepare the rest of your ingredients. Finely chop the cilantro and the green parts of your scallions, and then zest and squeeze juice from the fresh lime. Beat the egg in a small bowl, and add it into a large mixing bowl, along with the ground chicken, chili flakes, green onions, cilantro, sesame seeds, ginger, fish sauce, lime juice, brown sugar, and lime zest. Once the quinoa has cooked, add it into this mixing bowl, as well, and combine all the ingredients.

4. If your mixture looks a little soggy, you can remedy that by adding in some of the gluten-free all-purpose flour you have to absorb the extra water. Once it looks to be an appropriate consistency, begin to hand-roll the ground chicken and quinoa mixture into small, walnut-sized spheres.

5. Place the meatballs onto your baking sheet, making sure to leave sufficient space between each sphere. Bake them in the oven for about 18–20 minutes until all sides of the meatballs are

golden brown. Make sure the meatballs have been cooked all the way through before removing them from the oven.

6. While the meatballs are baking, begin making your teriyaki sauce. Heat a small saucepan over medium to high heat and add the rice vinegar, soy sauce, garlic-infused oil, crushed ginger, brown sugar, water, and sesame oil. On the side, dissolve the cornstarch into a little bit of warm water, and add it into the pot. Stir all the ingredients together and then leave the sauce to simmer slightly. Stir occasionally, allowing the teriyaki sauce to thicken for another 2–3 minutes. Give the sauce a taste, and add more rice wine vinegar or brown sugar if you would like. Once the sauce has thickened, remove it from heat and set aside.

7. Serve the meatballs on a plate or platter and garnish the top with a sprinkle of chopped green onions and some sesame seeds. Drizzle the teriyaki sauce over the top of the dish or serve on the side. Enjoy!

Lemon Coconut Cupcakes

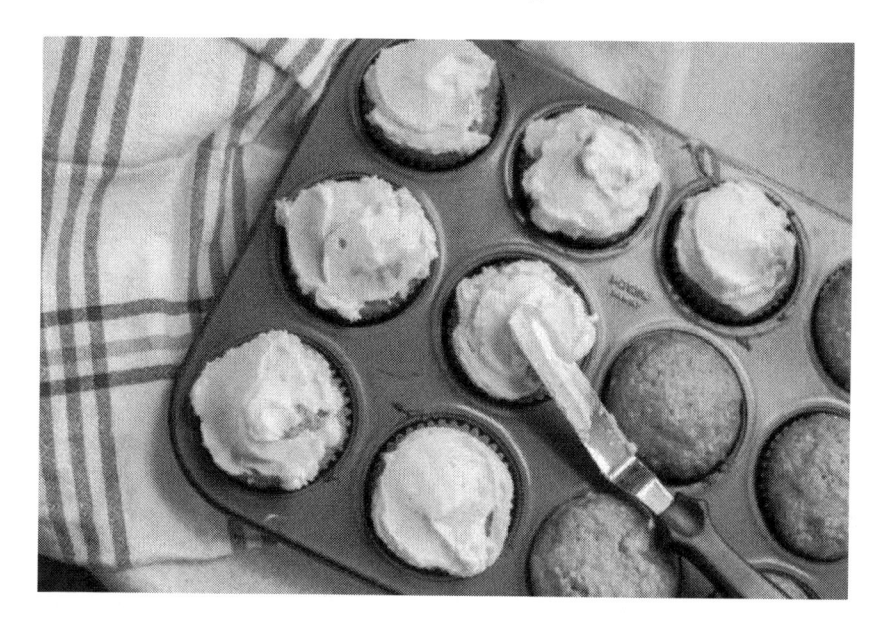

Cupcakes may be more of a dessert than a day-to-day snack but since these are low-FODMAP cupcakes, we can eat them with fewer regrets. Still, these cupcakes are full of sugar, so please make sure not to consume more than the recommended serving, which is just one cupcake so that you can continue enjoying treats like these for the rest of your long, healthy life! This recipe combines two classic flavors, and it takes only 25 minutes of prep time.

What You Will Need:

For the Cupcakes
- 1 muffin tin with at least 12 spots
- 1 and ½ cup of gluten-free all-purpose flour
- 1 large mixing bowl
- 1 hand beater or stand-alone mixer

- 1 small mixing bowl
- 115 g of olive oil spread (or dairy-free butter)
- 2 eggs
- 2 and ½ tbsp of lemon juice
- ½ cup of coconut yogurt
- ½ tsp of salt
- 1 tbsp of lemon zest
- 1 cup of white sugar
- ½ tsp of guar gum
- 1 tsp vanilla extract

Icing
- 100 g of olive oil spread (or dairy-free butter)
- 1 and ½ tbsp of lemon juice
- 1 and ½ cup of powdered sugar (confectioners sugar)

Low-FODMAP Shopping Tips:
- Choose a pure gluten-free flour that contains no chickpea/garbanzo flour, coconut flour, soy flour, lentil flour, amaranth flour, or lupin flour.
- Try to use fresh lemon juice and fresh lemon zest.
- You will likely find guar gum in your grocery store's gluten-free foods section because it is used primarily in gluten-free baking. This ingredient will help your gluten-free flour stick together and will allow the cupcakes to rise nicely.
- In this case, swapping out the coconut yogurt for another lactose-free yogurt is not an ideal option because your cupcakes will then lack the coconut flavor to compliment the lemon flavor. Choose a coconut yogurt that contains no inulin and no high-FODMAP sweeteners like fructose, high

fructose corn syrup, fructose glucose syrup, fruit juice, honey, or agave syrup. Also, check to make sure your coconut yogurt is pure and contains no high-FODMAP fruits.

Method:
1. Begin by preheating your oven to 355°F and greasing 12 spots in your muffin tin.

2. Start by combining the gluten-free all-purpose flour and guar gum—the dry ingredients. Then, mix in the salt, lemon zest, and baking powder. Mix everything well and then set the mixing bowl aside.

3. Now, take your room-temperature olive oil spread or dairy-free spread and mix it with all the white sugar in your large mixing bowl until they are combined well. Then, whisk in your eggs and vanilla extract and, once that mixture is smooth, add in the lemon juice. Blend these ingredients using whatever machine you have for this task. Using a spatula or large spoon will work as well but may take longer.

4. Then, add in small amounts of the dry ingredients from your small mixing bowl and small amounts of the coconut yogurt into the large mixing bowl. Keep alternating ingredients, and make sure to begin and end this process by adding in the dry mixture. Blend this until it is just combined.

5. Now, you can pour (or scoop using a ¼ cup measuring cup) the batter into the 12 spots that you greased on the baking pan earlier. Make sure to split the batter as evenly as possible to avoid overfilling a spot.

6. Place the muffin tin on the center tray in the oven. Bake the cupcakes for not more than 25 minutes. The cupcakes are done when their tops have a golden-brown color and a toothpick or fork comes out of the cupcakes completely clean.

7. If you would like to ice the cupcakes, begin making the icing while the cupcakes are baking in the oven.

8. In a small mixing bowl, combine your room-temperature olive oil spread or dairy-free butter with powdered sugar, making sure to add the powdered sugar slowly to the dairy-free spread as you combine them. Mix this with the lemon juice until the icing is smooth.

9. Once the cupcakes are fully done baking, pull the tin out of the oven and set it aside, so the cupcakes can cool. Once they have completely cooled, you can ice the cupcakes with a knife. Enjoy!

TIP: Please do not eat more than 1 cupcake serving, as there is a great amount of sugar used in this recipe. The cupcakes taste best on the day they are baked, so we encourage you to share them with friends or family! However, if this recipe is all for you, consider halving the ingredients and then storing the extra cupcakes in an airtight container in the pantry. Heat the leftover cupcakes in the microwave for 5 seconds before you eat them, so they will be fresh and fluffy again. Take care and enjoy!

Salted Caramel Pumpkin Seeds

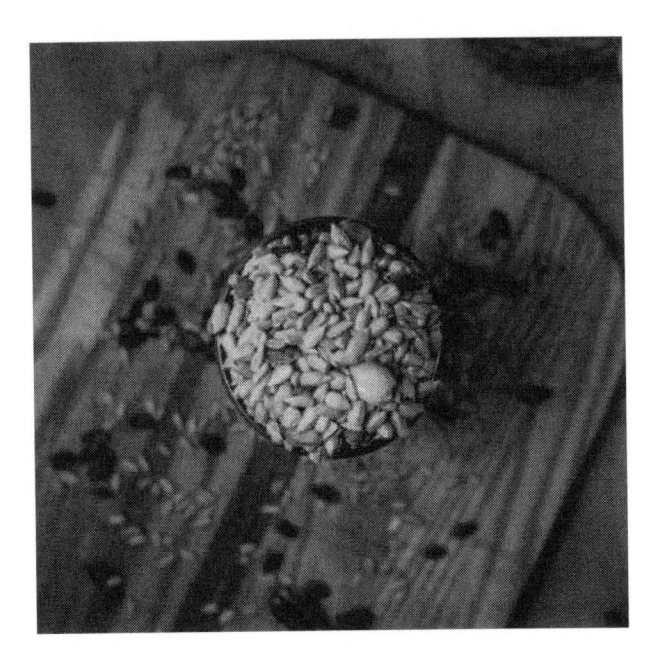

These tasty pumpkin seeds are a great snack to nibble on throughout the day because the seeds themselves are so healthy and nutritious. These seeds also make the perfect toppings for fruit bowls, oatmeal, or ice cream! The prep time for the seeds is only 5 minutes and this recipe yields 16 servings to last you through a couple of weeks.

<u>What You Will Need:</u>
- 1 large mixing bowl
- 1 baking tray
- ⅛ tsp of ground nutmeg
- 2 cups of pumpkin seeds
- ½ tsp of ground ginger
- 2 and ½ tbsp white sugar
- 1 and ½ tbsp of olive oil spread or dairy-free butter

- ¼ tsp of ground cinnamon
- 3 and ½ tbsp of brown sugar
- ½ tsp of rock salt
- 2 tsp of water

Method:
1. Begin by preheating your oven to 350° F and greasing or laying baking paper across your baking tray.

2. Mix your pumpkin seeds, ginger, nutmeg, 1 and ½ tbsp of white sugar, cinnamon, and water in a large mixing bowl. Make sure to add the exact amount of water specified because you want the spice mixture to stick well to the seeds and not runoff.

3. After the seeds are all fully coated with the spices and sugar, pour them into your baking tray, and spread them out so that they all bake evenly. Put the tray in the oven for about 20–25 minutes and stir the seeds once during this time. Remove the seeds from the oven once the seeds have a slight golden color and are crunchy.

4. You can leave the seeds as is and snack on them straight after they have baked, or you can create a salted caramel sauce to add more flavor to the pumpkin seeds. Just as the seeds finish baking, melt your dairy-free spread in a small saucepan over medium heat. Mix in the brown sugar, rock salt, and the remaining white sugar. Allow this mixture to heat for about 2 minutes until it takes

on a deep golden color, and lower the heat under the saucepan. Pour the baked seeds into the saucepan, and mix them so that they are evenly coated with the salted caramel mixture. Once all the sauce is on the pumpkin seeds, pour them back into the baking tray, and allow the seeds to cool and the salted caramel sauce to harden.

5. Serve these as a topping for some other food or eat them on their own. Enjoy!

Falafel

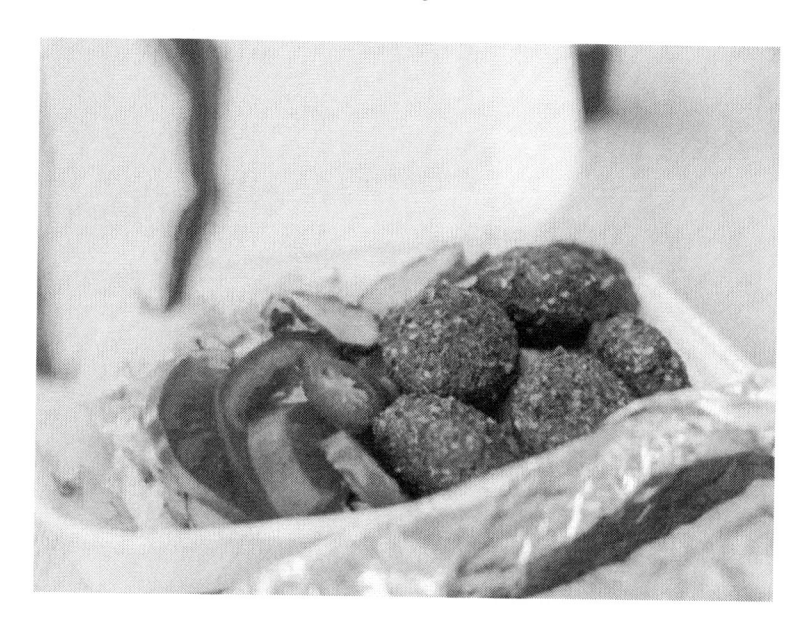

These falafel are a great vegan snack option and are also great for people who prefer savory over sweet snacks. You can change the snack you eat by serving the falafels with a different side each time. We recommend that you give the homemade garlic-infused mayonnaise recipe a try. It is provided at the end of this recipe. This snack takes only about 25 minutes of total cooking time and yields 5 servings of 4 falafels each.

What You Will Need:
- 1 blender or food processor
- 1 large frying pan
- 1 tbsp of olive oil
- 1 baking tray
- 2 medium-sized carrots
- 4 tbsp gluten-free all-purpose flour

- 1 cup of canned chickpeas
- 1 cup of leeks (green part only)
- Salt and pepper
- 1 cup of cooked brown rice
- 1 large lime
- 1 cup of fresh parsley
- 1 tbsp of garlic-infused oil
- 1 tsp of paprika
- ¾ tsp of ground cumin

Low-FODMAP Shopping Tips:
- Buy garlic-infused oil that is free of garlic bits. We want to capture the garlic flavor without adding in the high-FODMAP fructans from the garlic itself.
- The green tips of the leek are the low-FODMAP part, so buy leeks with long green stems.
- Choose a pure gluten-free flour that contains no chickpea/garbanzo flour, coconut flour, soy flour, lentil flour, amaranth flour, or lupin flour.
- Use a fresh lime because you will be taking the zest and juicing it.
- Chickpeas can be high in FODMAP in higher quantities, but you will stay within the diet guidelines if you stick to the suggested serving size and use canned chickpeas. The oligosaccharides from the chickpeas will leak into the brine inside the can and will make the chickpeas themselves much lower in FODMAPs.

Method:
1. Begin by preparing your vegetables to cook. Peel and grate your carrots, zest, and juice the lime, roughly chop the green leaves of the leek, and

roughly chop the fresh parsley. Then, completely drain and rinse the canned chickpeas.

2. Place all of these ingredients in the food processor in no particular order. Begin blending the ingredients into a smooth paste, and add a splash of water to the blender if the mixture is too dry to combine well.

3. At this point, stir in your gluten-free all-purpose flour so that the mixture is at the right consistency to handle and shape.

4. We have provided you with two options for cooking:

    - Cooking in the Oven: This method is ideal if you like crispy falafels and don't have the time to watch over them closely as they cook. Preheat your oven to 375° F and prepare your baking tray by lightly greasing it or covering it with baking paper. Scoop out one tablespoon at a time of the falafel mixture, and use your clean hands to shape the mixture into small patties. Lay all the falafel patties on the baking tray, making sure to keep sufficient space between each of them. Lightly coat the tops of each patty in olive oil, and it's ready for the oven. Set your baking timer for 12 minutes. When the alarm sounds, flip the patties and leave them for another 12 minutes. Remove from the oven once the falafels are golden brown on either side.

- Cooking in the frying pan: This method is ideal if you like softer falafels and if you have the time to mind the falafels as they cook individually. Grease your large frying pan with about a tablespoon of olive oil and heat it using medium-high flame over the stove. Scoop out one tablespoon at a time of the falafel mixture, and use your clean hands to shape the mixture into small patties. Lay all the falafel patties on the frying pan and cook each side of each patty for about 2–3 minutes until everything is cooked through and has turned a nice golden-brown color. You will likely need to cook the falafels in several batches, so make sure to turn down the heat or add more oil as needed. Place the finished falafels onto a paper towel to help any excess oil to drain.

5. As the falafels finish baking or after you have finished cooking in the frying pan, you can start making the homemade garlic-infused mayonnaise.

6. Use vegan mayonnaise, and make sure it has no onions or garlic in it. Mix a small amount of lemon or lime juice with the mayonnaise, garlic-infused oil, and a sprinkle of black pepper. Mix

these ingredients, and add more or less of any of these based on your taste and preferences.

7. Serve your falafel patties on a large plate with garlic-infused mayonnaise on the side. Enjoy!

Chapter 7: Meatless Meals

Vegetarian Recipes

Unique Vegetable Pizza

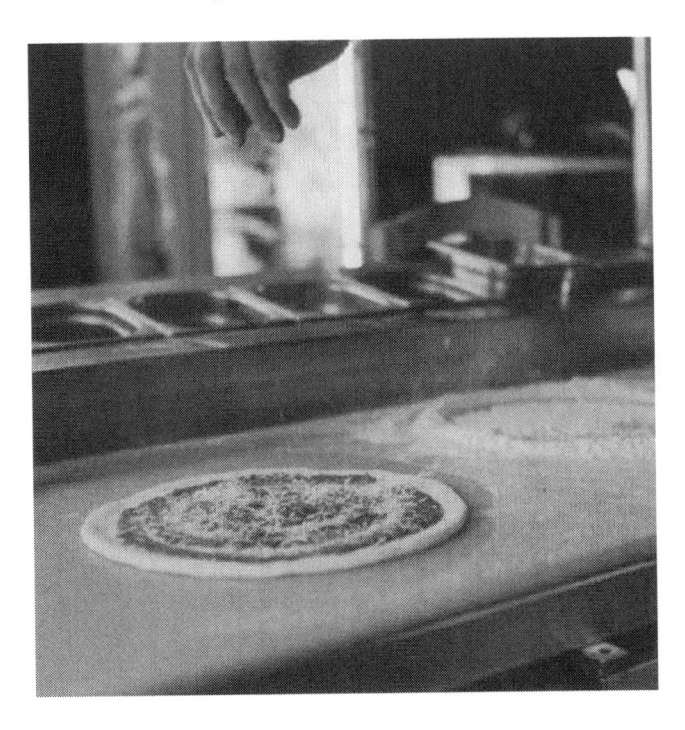

Pizza is a classic favorite dish, and now, you can make a vegetarian pizza that is also a low-FODMAP meal! Although this recipe is lengthier with a 45-minute prep time and 15-minute cooking time, it yields 4 delicious servings and is most definitely worth the wait. This particular recipe incorporates pumpkin, sweet potatoes, capsicum, and spinach to create the perfect blend of flavors in pizza form!

What You Will Need:
- 1 oven tray or pan
- 1 stick blender/food processor
- 1 cup of baby spinach
- 1 roasting tray or pan
- 2 gluten-free pizza bases
- 1 cup of mozzarella cheese (OR a vegan soy-based cheese)
- 1 and ½ tsp of dried oregano
- 4 tbsp of tomato paste
- 1 tbsp of garlic-infused oil
- 1 large carrot
- 3 tbsp of fresh chives
- 2 tsp of fresh thyme
- 240 g of Japanese pumpkin (OR sweet potato or buttercup squash)
- 1 handful of fresh baby basil leaves
- 2 red bell peppers
- 1 tbsp of rice bran, sunflower, OR canola oil (natural oils)
- 270 g of sweet potato
- Salt and pepper

Low-FODMAP Shopping Tips:
- A mozzarella is a low-FODMAP option, but if you choose a vegan cheese, check to make sure it contains no garlic or onion.
- Buy garlic-infused oil that is free of garlic bits. We want to capture the garlic flavor without adding in the high-FODMAP fructans from the garlic itself.
- Choose a gluten-free pizza base that is free of high-FODMAP ingredients, such as apple fiber,

inulin, coconut flour, soy flour, besan/garbanzo flour, lupin flour, and amaranth flour.
- Sweet potatoes are low in FODMAP only in small servings, so try not to exceed the suggested serving size listed above. If you would like to be extra cautious, you can substitute carrots, regular potatoes, or parsnip in place of the sweet potatoes.

Method:

1. Begin by preheating your oven to 390°F.

2. First, peel and then chop the pumpkin and sweet potatoes into medium cubes and lay them all over a roasting tray. Add deseeded and sliced red bell peppers to the tray, along with a drizzle of natural oil. Dust the veggies with some pepper and salt before baking for at least 20 minutes. Add 10 minutes to the baking time if needed or until the veggies become crispy. You may need to toss the veggies once or twice while they bake to ensure that they roast evenly.

3. Add 1 tbsp of water to a microwave-safe bowl, peel and cut the carrots, also in the same size, and add them to the bowl. Cover the bowl and microwave the carrots for 2–3 minutes until they soften. Drain out the extra water and puree the soft carrots in a blender. In a separate bowl, mix the tomato paste and the carrot puree you just created.

4. Cover your pizza bases with the tomato and carrot mixture and then season it with oregano. Spread the baked veggies evenly over the pizza bases and top with grated cheese.

5. Bake the bases for 15 minutes in the preheated oven. Or bake them until their hues change to a golden brown.

6. Remove baking trays and sprinkle salt, pepper, chopped spinach, baby basil leaves, thyme, and chives over the hot pizzas. Finally, drizzle garlic-infused oil over the pizza and enjoy!

Pumpkin Carrot Risotto

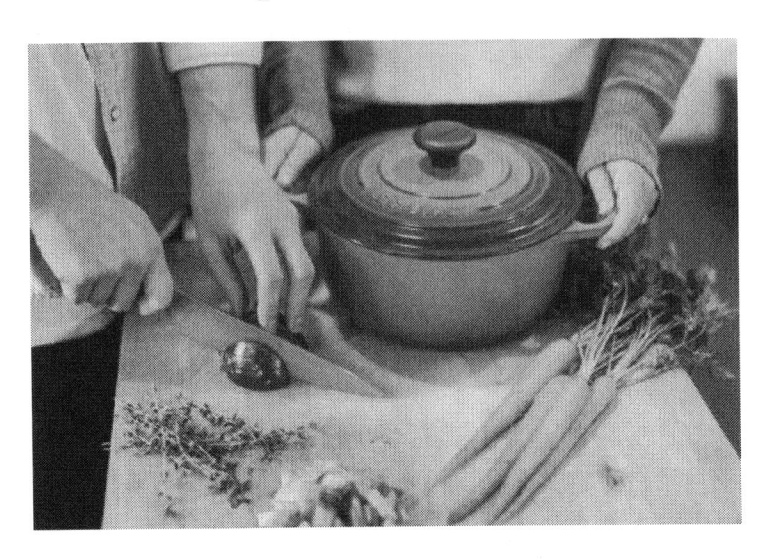

This delicious risotto combines flavors to create fresh comfort food. On its own, this dish is the perfect vegetarian meal. However, if you prefer extra protein, you can pair this dish with some pan-fried fish. This recipe cooks in 35 minutes and yields 4 servings.

What You Will Need:
- 1 roasting tray or pan
- 1 large saucepan
- 240 g of Japanese pumpkin (OR sweet potato or buttercup squash)
- 2 and ½ of tbsp lemon juice
- 1 and ½ of cup uncooked risotto rice
- ½ cup of leeks (only use the green tips)
- 1 tbsp of garlic-infused oil
- 4 cups of a low-FODMAP vegetable stock
- 4 cups of spinach leaves
- 2 large carrots

- Salt and pepper
- 2 tsp of lemon zest
- 3 tbsp of fresh cilantro
- 1 tbsp of olive oil spread OR dairy-free butter
- 1 tbsp of olive oil
- 50 g of parmesan cheese (OR vegan soy-based cheese)

Low-FODMAP Shopping Tips:
- Buy garlic-infused oil that is free of garlic bits. We want to capture the garlic flavor without adding in the high-FODMAP fructans from the garlic itself.
- Parmesan cheese is low in FODMAP, but if you choose a vegan soy-based cheese, make sure it contains no onion, garlic, or coconut flour.
- Choose a vegetable stock that contains no onion or garlic.
- The green tips of the leek are the low-FODMAP part, so buy leeks with long green stems.
- Choose medium-grain risotto rice because it will help bring out a creamy flavor and taste.
- Try to use juice and zest from a fresh lemon.

Method:
1. Begin by preheating your oven to 390° F.

2. Peel the skin off the carrots and pumpkin. Chop them into small, even-sized pieces and distribute them evenly on a roasting tray, coating with olive oil. Dust some pepper and salt, according to your preference. Bake the veggies for 25 minutes at most or until they begin to look soft and the color

is golden brown. Make sure to toss the veggies a couple of times as they cook.

3. Add your dairy-free spread and garlic-infused oil into a large saucepan and cook roughly chopped leeks in the pan for 2 minutes over medium heat. Add your uncooked risotto rice to the pot and stir for a minute. Pour the vegetable stock, gradually (a half cup at each time) until the rice cooks and absorbs all the liquid. Lower the heat as the rice cooks more and more to avoid any of it sticking to the bottom of the pot.

4. As the rice finishes cooking, add in your shredded spinach, salt, pepper, lemon juice, and lemon zest. Finally, stir in the baked pumpkin and carrot pieces and top with chopped fresh cilantro and the cheese of your choice.

5. Serve in a bowl while hot and enjoy!

Fennel Carrot Soup

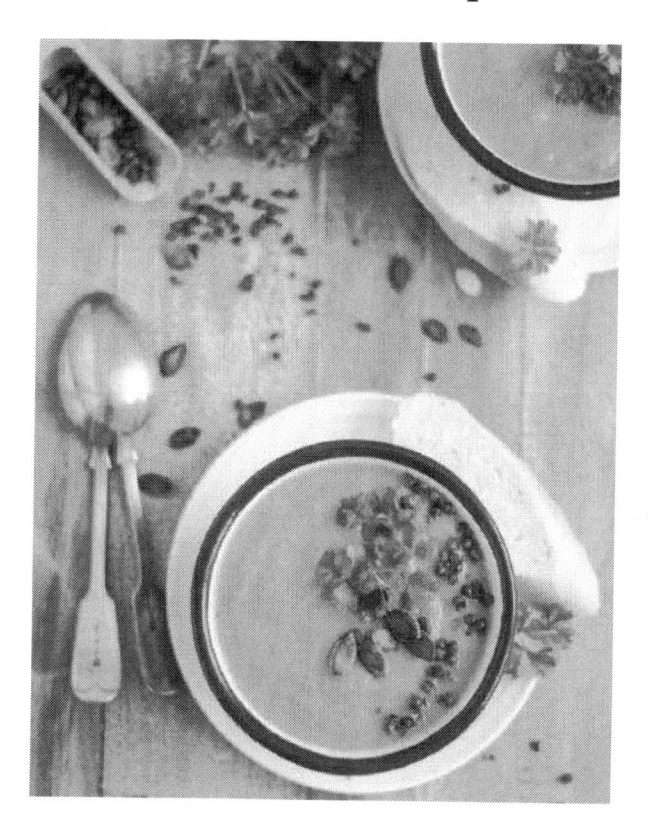

This dish has a unique flavor and aromatic taste. The soup pairs nicely with a piece of crunchy bread and make the perfect meal. Although the soup can take a while to cook, the preparation takes only 10 minutes and the recipe serves 4! As a bonus, this soup also freezes well. You can freeze leftovers and reheat as needed in a microwave or over the stove until it is warm.

What You Will Need:
- 1 large saucepan
- 1 blender/food processor
- 2 large carrots

- 200 g of sweet potatoes
- 340 g of regular potatoes
- ½ cup of leeks (only use the green tips)
- 3 cups of a low-FODMAP vegetable stock
- 1 tbsp of garlic-infused oil
- 1 tbsp of olive oil spread OR dairy-free butter
- 1 and ½ tbsp of fresh cilantro
- ½ cup of a low-FODMAP milk
- 1 tbsp of olive oil
- 8 slices of a low-FODMAP bread
- Salt and pepper

Low-FODMAP Shopping Tips:
- Buy garlic-infused oil that is free of garlic bits. We want to capture the garlic flavor without adding in the high-FODMAP fructans from the garlic itself.
- The green tips of the leek are the low-FODMAP part, so buy leeks with long green stems.
- Buy low-FODMAP bread that contains no chickpea/garbanzo flour, coconut flour, soy flour, amaranth flour, or lupin flour. Also, try to avoid ingredients like concentrated fruit juices, pear juice, apple juice, inulin, apple fiber, high-fructose corn syrup, or honey. Wheat sourdough bread can be a good low-FODMAP option.
- Sweet potatoes are low in FODMAP only in small servings, so try not to exceed the suggested serving size listed above. If you would like to be extra cautious, you can substitute carrots, regular potatoes, or parsnip in place of the sweet potatoes.
- Choose a low-FODMAP vegetable stock that is free of onions and garlic.

Method:
1. Begin by thinly slicing the green tips of the leeks. Peel the potatoes, carrots, and sweet potatoes and then chop them into small chunks.

2. Warm a large saucepan using a low flame, and pour both the olive oil and garlic-infused oil. When it's warm enough, cook the sliced leeks, stirring occasionally. They cook fast—about a minute—so watch out. After this, add the potatoes, sweet potatoes, and carrots into the saucepan and cook on low for about 5 minutes. Continue stirring the contents of the saucepan.

3. Turn the flame under the saucepan to medium, and add the vegetable stock. Allow the soup to boil and then cover the saucepan. Let it simmer for not more than 15 minutes or until the veggies are soft.

4. While the soup is simmering, melt the dairy-free spread in a frying pan, where you heat the fennel seeds for about a minute while stirring. Add in freshly chopped cilantro and stir together for another minute. Add this fennel and cilantro mixture to the soup.

5. Pour the soup out of the large saucepan, and allow it to cool for about 10 minutes once the vegetables are fully tender. Then, pour the soup into a blender and process until the soup is smooth and looks more or less homogenous.

6. Pour the soup mixture back into a saucepan and begin reheating it over a low flame. Mix in your low-FODMAP milk and make sure to season with salt and pepper.

7. Top the soup with fresh cilantro and a side of lightly toasted low-FODMAP bread. Enjoy!

Vegan Recipes

Lentil and Rice Bowl

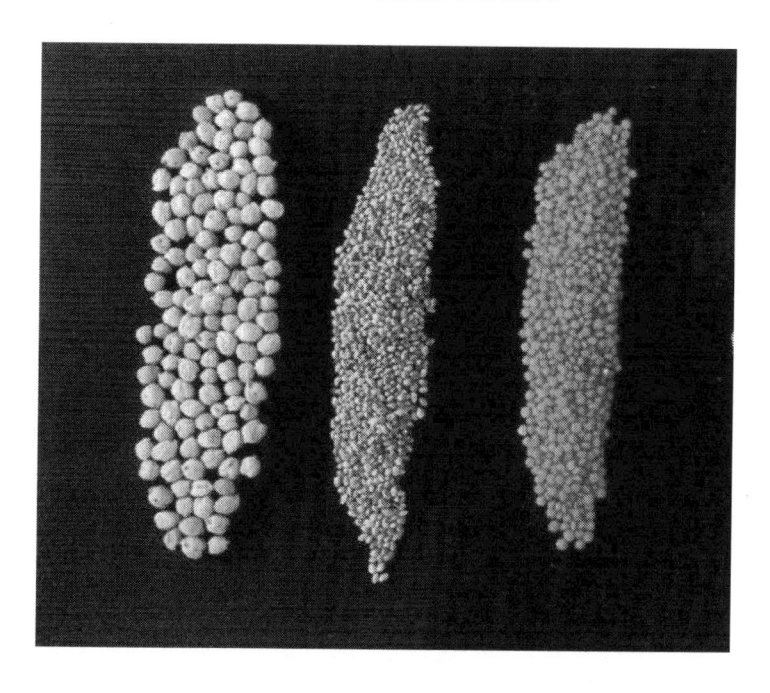

This vegan bowl is full of flavor from deliciously prepared veggies, rice, lentils, and seeds. The rice can take up to 30 minutes to cook but the preparation for the bowl takes only 15 minutes! This nourishing bowl is a perfect blend of nutrients and this recipe yields 4 servings.

What You Will Need:
- 1 large saucepan
- 1 roasting pan or tray
- 2 cups of frozen edamame beans
- 1 small saucepan
- 1 large frying pan

- 1 blender/food processor
- 400 g of canned lentils
- Salt and pepper
- 3 cups of low-FODMAP vegetable stock
- 240 g of Japanese pumpkin (OR sweet potato or buttercup squash)
- 1 tbsp of olive oil
- 1 and ½ cups of uncooked long-grain brown rice
- ½ tsp of smoked paprika
- ¼ cup of green onions/scallions (only use green part)
- 3 large carrots
- Juice of 0.5 large lime
- 1 and ½ cups of baby spinach leaves
- 1 red chili - mild
- 1 pinch of chili powder
- ½ cup + 3 tbsp of fresh cilantro
- 2 tsp of garlic-infused oil
- 1 tsp of ground cumin
- 3 tbsp of lightly toasted pumpkin seeds

Low-FODMAP Shopping Tips:
- The high-FODMAP oligosaccharides in lentils dissipate into the canned liquid, so the lentils themselves become low-FODMAP. Make sure to drain and rinse the lentils well before using them
- Buy garlic-infused oil that is free of garlic bits. We want to capture the garlic flavor without adding in the high-FODMAP fructans from the garlic itself.
- Choose a pure chili powder that is not mixed with other ingredients, including high-FODMAP garlic powder.

- Choose a vegetable stock that contains no onion or garlic.

Method:
1. Begin by preheating your oven to 390° F.

2. Place the rice into a large saucepan over a medium flame, add in your vegetable stock, and bring the contents of the saucepan to a rolling boil. When it has started to boil, cover the pot, and reduce the flame. Allow the rice to simmer for 20 minutes. Add another 10 minutes when the water has not fully evaporated.

3. Peel and cut the pumpkin and carrots to your desired size; ideally, they have to be small pieces. Coat the pumpkin and carrot chunks in olive oil, salt, and smoked paprika, and place them in a roasting tray. Bake them for up to 30 minutes until they appear golden brown, making sure to toss the veggies once as they cook.

4. Roughly chop the chilies, spinach, and green onions, making sure to deseed the chilies first. Place them in the blender, along with garlic-infused oil, ½ cup cilantro, and 3 tbsp of water. Blend the ingredients into a chunky paste and then stir in with the brown rice while it cooks. Once the rice is finished, let it stand for 10 minutes and then fluff the rice, adding some salt and pepper according to your preference.

5. Set a frying pan over medium flame on the stove. Drain and rinse the canned lentils and add them to the pan. Add the cumin and chili powder, as well as the quarter cup of water to the pan and simmer for a maximum of 5 minutes or until the water has been incorporated into the lentils. Remove the lentils from the heat and place them on the side. Add some lime juice and some more salt and pepper, if you wish

6. Boil the frozen edamame beans in a saucepan until they are tender.

7. In a serving bowl, plate the spiced rice and lentils, and top it with edamame, roasted veggies, pumpkin seeds, and the remaining cilantro. Enjoy!

Kale and Olive Pasta

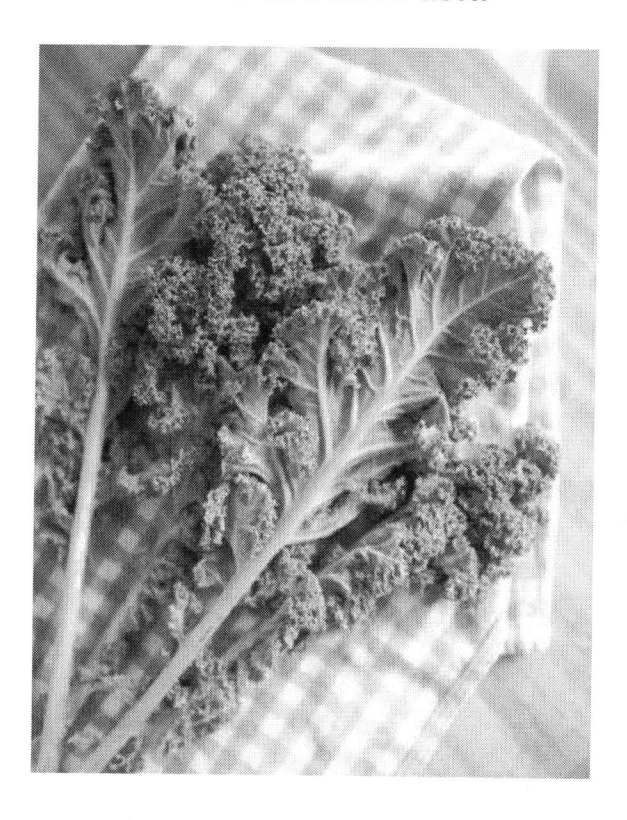

This recipe will help you create a meal that is low in FODMAP and also fits into a whole-food, plant-based diet! If you have been worried about maintaining proper nutrition with a diet that is vegan and is low in FODMAP, then this is the perfect recipe for you! You will get plenty of protein from the green lentils and will have enough grains and greens to keep your stomach full and happy. This dish will take you under 15 minutes to cook and will leave you with one full serving of delicious pasta!

What You Will Need:

- 1 large saucepan
- 1 large frying pan
- 70 g of gluten-free pasta uncooked
- 46 g of canned green lentils
- 2 full handfuls of kale (you can use more or less depending on your tastes)
- 2-3 common tomatoes
- 1 sundried tomato
- 2 tbsp of pumpkin seeds
- Salt and pepper
- 1 tbsp of pitted black olives
- 1 tbsp of uncooked tomato puree
- 1 tsp of garlic-infused oil
- 1 tsp of balsamic vinegar

Low-FODMAP Shopping Tips:
- Buy garlic-infused oil that is free of garlic bits. We want to capture the garlic flavor without adding in the high-FODMAP fructans from the garlic itself
- Choose a pure gluten-free pasta to avoid high-FODMAP ingredients like wheat, soy flour, amaranth flour, lupin flour, or inulin.
- The high-FODMAP oligosaccharides in lentils dissipate into the canned liquid, so the lentils themselves become low in FODMAP. Make sure to drain and rinse the lentils well before using them.

Method:
1. Begin by heating water in your large saucepan. Once it comes to a boil, add in a little salt for flavor, and then place your gluten-free pasta. Let the pasta cook according to the package directions.

2. Place your large frying pan over a medium flame and pour in your sunflower seeds so that they begin to toast. This should be done while the seeds and your pan are dry. Once the seeds begin to give off a nutty aroma and start popping in the pan, add your drained and rinsed lentils. Stir the seeds and lentils together for a minute or two and then add chopped kale and sliced tomatoes to the pan. You might need to add some water to the pan so that the kale reduces as it cooks and doesn't burn.

3. Once the kale has begun to cook down, stir in your finely chopped sundried tomato, black olives, balsamic vinegar, garlic-infused oil, and tomato puree and let everything cook together. As you stir the sauce, add in little bits of water if you need to thin down the sauce or help it cooks. Heat and stir the sauce until it begins to smush together.

4. Your sauce should be done by the time your pasta is done cooking in the pot. At this point, add the cooked pasta into the large frying pan with the sauce and stir everything together to combine it evenly.

5. To finish, serve your pasta dish in a large bowl with a sprinkle of pepper or salt to your liking. Enjoy!

Chinese Noodle Soup

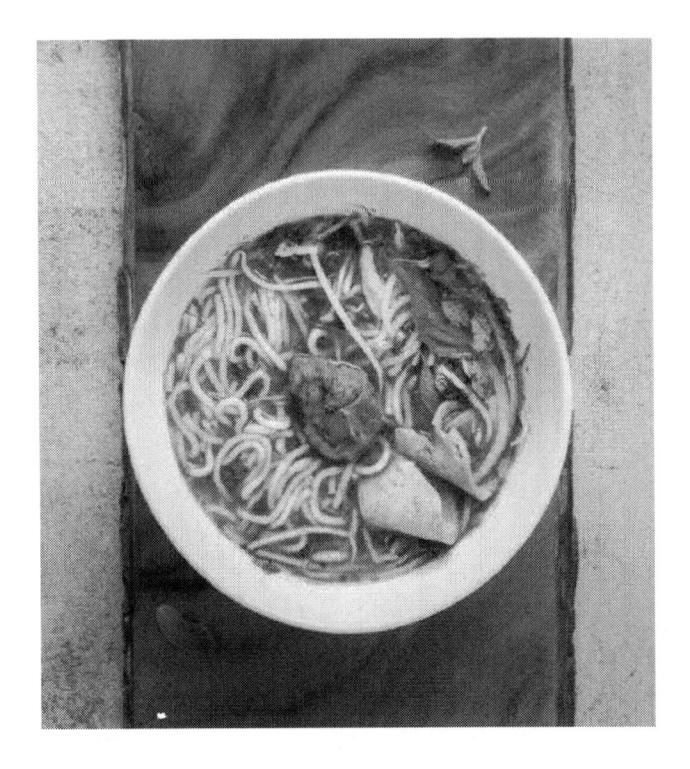

This soup is not only nourishing but is extremely gentle on your body, so it is the perfect meal to eat if you have been experiencing a particularly nasty IBS flare-up. This recipe is also super easy and quick to prepare, so it is ideal if you are not feeling your best! In only 8 minutes, you will have a large serving of the best noodle soup with tofu and tomatoes.

What You Will Need:
- 1 large saucepan
- 100 g of firm tofu
- 1 large tomato
- 1 sheet of Nori (seaweed sheet)

- 1 tbsp sesame oil
- 2 cups of a low-FODMAP vegetable stock
- 1 full nest of rice noodles
- ¼ tsp of turmeric
- 2 tbsp of green onions/scallions (only use green part)
- 2 tsp of ginger root
- 1 tbsp soy sauce
- 1 tsp corn starch or cornflour
- 1 tsp miso paste

Low-FODMAP Shopping Tips:
- Nori (seaweed) sheets should be stocked in normal supermarkets but will be abundant in your local Asian market.
- If you want to be extra cautious, you can swap normal soy sauce for its gluten-free version to make sure it is low in FODMAP.
- Choose firm tofu so that you can be sure it is low in FODMAP.

Method:
1. Chop your tofu into small, bite-sized chunks, and chop the Nori sheet into small flakes. Peel the ginger root and then make sure to dice both the tomato and the ginger root finely.

2. Set your saucepan over medium heat, heat half the sesame oil in the pot, and then add in your tofu chunks. Place your turmeric powder, finely chopped ginger, and half of your soy sauce over the tofu. Once it has begun to warm up, stir in

your miso paste and finely diced tomatoes. Add salt and pepper to taste.

3. As this tofu mixture continues to heat up, pour in the vegetable stock and break the rice noodles into it. Let the noodles soften in the vegetable stock for about 2–3 minutes and then sprinkle in the Nori flakes.

4. In a separate small bowl, mix your corn starch or cornflour with about 2 tbsp of water. Pour this mixture into the noodle soup that you are cooking in your pot, and begin to stir the soup very fast. Continue to stir as the soup begins to thicken.

5. Serve in a bowl. Pour the rest of the sesame oil and soy sauce over the soup. Finally, season the soup with your green onions and black pepper and enjoy!

Indian Spinach Tofu Curry

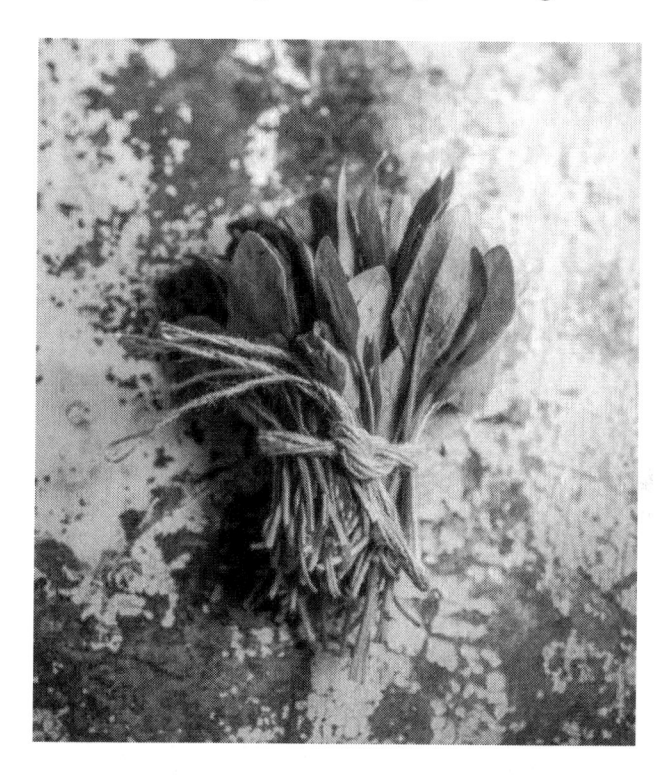

Indian vegan food is rare to come by, not to mention Indian low-FODMAP vegan food. But, that's exactly what this recipe delivers, and it is quite delicious! This recipe is adapted from an Indian classic dish called Palak Paneer which is loaded with garlic, onions, and more spinach than you can imagine. It is also full of dairy as paneer is a sort of Indian cheese. This recipe is free of high-FODMAP triggers and still offers a delicious punch of unique flavors packed into a nutritious meal! You can pair this curry with low-FODMAP rice or gluten-free chapati (stick to an appropriate serving size for both) to complete the meal! In total, this recipe takes a total of 40 minutes to cook, but it is completely worth it because it will leave you with 2 full servings that will leave you wanting more.

What You Will Need:
- 1 small to a medium-sized mixing bowl
- 1 large frying pan
- 1 food processor/blender
- 200 g of firm tofu
- 1 tsp of cumin seeds
- 3 small-medium sized tomatoes
- 2 inches of ginger root
- 2 cups of baby spinach
- 3 and ½ tbsp of coconut cream
- ½ tsp of turmeric powder
- ½ tsp of pure asafoetida
- 1 tsp of cumin powder
- 2 tsp of garam masala
- 2 tsp of garlic-infused oil
- Salt, pepper, and cayenne pepper
- 5 large leaves of chard
- 2 tsp of sesame oil
- 4 tbsp of green onions/scallions (only use green part)
- 2 tsp of soy sauce
- 2 tbsp of rice bran, sunflower, OR canola oil (natural oils)

Low-FODMAP Shopping Tips:
- Choose firm tofu so that you can be sure it is low in FODMAP. Although the ingredients list above suggests 200 g of firm tofu for the entire recipe, you can add more protein to your meal by using up to 160 g of tofu per serving.

- If you want to be extra cautious, you can swap normal soy sauce for its gluten-free version to make sure it is low in FODMAP.
- Asafoetida powder is an Indian spice that packs savory dishes and curries with an extra punch by adding in garlic and onion flavors. Choose a pure asafoetida powder so that you get a stronger flavor with less of the spice and avoid hidden high-FODMAP ingredients in your spice.
- Buy garlic-infused oil that is free of garlic bits. We want to capture the garlic flavor without adding in the high-FODMAP fructans from the garlic itself.
- Spices like garam masala should be available at your local grocery store but will be abundant in your local Indian Market store. There you can also purchase cumin seeds, cumin powder, asafoetida powder, and turmeric powder.

Method:
1. Start by chopping the firm tofu into bite-sized pieces and mixing the tofu cubes with soy sauce and turmeric powder in your mixing bowl. Then prepare your ginger and green onions by finely chopping them. Chop the tomatoes as well with less precision since a small-piece size is not so essential for the tomatoes.

2. Place your frying pan over medium heat and pour your garam masala, asafoetida, and cumin seeds into the pan. Let the spices toast for a few seconds on the heated pan surface and then add in your natural oil so that the spices can fry. Let the spices and oil warm for one more minute before adding

the chopped ginger and green onion to the frying pan.

3. Remove the green onions from the pan once they begin to crisp up a little bit and place them to the side. Add the marinated tofu cubes into the same frying pan and cook the pieces until they have a golden-brown color all around. At this point, remove the tofu from the pan and set the pieces aside as well.

4. Now, add your crispy green onions to your food processor along with the tomatoes, baby spinach leaves, and roughly chopped chard leaves. Blend the ingredients until they create a sort of bright-green homogenous mixture.

5. Add some water to the mixture in the blender, and pour it all out into the hot frying pan. Heat this mixture on medium heat for about 10 minutes. You'll know the mixture is sufficiently cooked once it no longer has a "grassy" aroma or taste to it.

6. When this mixture has cooked for around 10 minutes, add cumin seeds, garlic-infused oil, sesame oil, and coconut cream to the pan. Season this new mixture with cayenne pepper, salt, and black pepper.

7. Add the golden-brown tofu pieces to the curry in the pan and let everything heat evenly.

8. Serve this curry over a bowl of fresh rice or next to a gluten-free chapati. Enjoy!

Spinach Eggplant Pasta

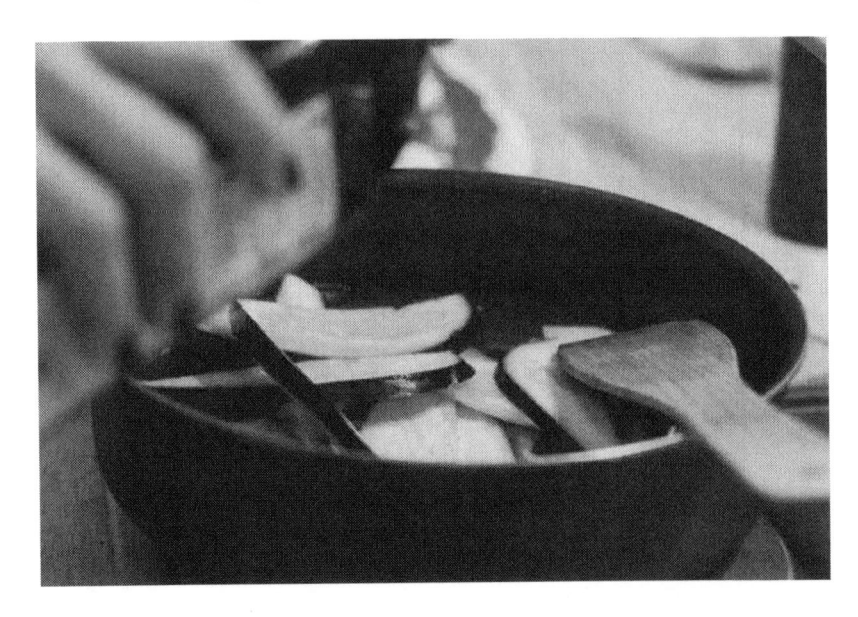

This pasta dish uses buckwheat pasta that gives a unique flavor and has a texture that is much more similar to pasta that is not gluten-free. You will feel as if you are having a high-FODMAP meal again without experiencing the negative digestive symptoms that accompany the meal. The buckwheat pasta is low in FODMAP only in small quantities, so make sure not to exceed the serving size listed below. If you would like to increase the ratio of pasta to veggie sauce in this recipe, consider switching to a different gluten-free pasta with a higher recommended serving size. This pasta dish recipe takes under 15 minutes to prepare and yields 1 full serving!

What You Will Need:
- 1 large saucepan
- 1 large frying pan
- 1 cup of uncooked buckwheat pasta

- 1 cup of baby spinach
- 1 tsp of olive oil
- 3 tbsp of uncooked tomato puree
- ½ of an eggplant
- Salt and pepper
- 2 tbsp of pine nuts
- 1 tsp of garlic-infused oil
- 2 tbsp of chives

Low-FODMAP Shopping Tips:
- Buy garlic-infused oil that is free of garlic bits. We want to capture the garlic flavor without adding in the high-FODMAP fructans from the garlic itself.
- If you decide not to use buckwheat pasta, choose a pure gluten-free pasta in its place, so you can avoid high-FODMAP ingredients like wheat, soy flour, amaranth flour, lupin flour, or inulin.

Method:
1. Begin by boiling some water for the pasta in a large saucepan. Place the pasta in the saucepan, along with a dash of salt or according to your preference. Cook the pasta according to the package instructions, though it generally shouldn't take longer than 10 minutes.

2. Place your frying pan over medium heat and begin to dry toast your pine nuts until they turn a warm golden color. While they are heating, chop up your eggplant into small, bite-sized cubes. Once toasted, set the pine nuts aside.

3. In the same heated pan, add your eggplant cubes and cook them dry in the pan over a high flame. As the eggplant is heating, sprinkle some salt over the pieces so that they begin to release some water and brown over. Now, you can add half of the garlic-infused oil and olive oil to the cooked eggplant. Stir fry the eggplant pieces in the oil until they are completely cooked and softened.

4. Bring the heat under the frying pan to low and add your tomato puree to the cooked eggplant cubes in the pan. Stir in your roughly chopped spinach, 1 tbsp of chives, and a tbsp or so of extra water. Allow this mixture to heat evenly, and let the spinach wilt.

5. At this point, transfer your cooked pasta to the sauce in the pan. Serve this pasta in a bowl and top it with the remaining garlic-infused oil, 1 tbsp of chives, and the dry toasted pine nuts. Enjoy!

Chapter 8: Why Is This Diet Not Working For Me?

I hope most of you were able to experience a significant reduction in your IBS symptoms and that you have moved on to personalizing and maintaining your diet. If you did not have this experience, there are several things about the way you might have proceeded with the diet that could be preventing you from enjoying reduced gut symptoms. There is also the chance that you completed this diet perfectly in all its phases and still did not see results. Regardless of which category you fall into, the following are some of the reasons you may not have seen significant results after following the low-FODMAP diet:

1. **Your gut is not overly sensitive to high-FODMAP foods:** Research has demonstrated that the low-FODMAP diet is extremely beneficial to people who have IBS with a sensitive gut but, as we all know, each body is extremely different. You can have severe IBS without being particularly sensitive to different foods. In this case, it is ideal to talk with a doctor about further treatment approaches. They may suggest ideas like talk therapy if you suffer from extreme stress or medication options if you have tried other methods and not seen a reduction of IBS symptoms. It may even be beneficial to you to go through and follow the diet one more time while you are practicing good stress management.

2. **You did not properly follow the guidelines of the diet:** As I prefaced at the beginning of the book, the low-FODMAP diet can be challenging to follow, especially if you are used to eating in large quantities or if you generally ingest a large amount of high-FODMAP foods. This diet requires focus and strict adherence to the guidelines, so for the low-FODMAP diet to be successful, you must follow through with each phase completely. It is also important to remember that even one "cheat" meal, where you eat high-FODMAP foods, can risk your positive results with the elimination phase.

   If you feel as if you did not give this diet a fair and sincere chance, it is still possible that the diet can work for you in the future. Take some time to refocus yourself and remember what you are trying to accomplish with the low-FODMAP diet—you want to see your IBS symptoms decrease! Try to meet with a dietary professional so that you can have better guidance the next time you follow this diet. Then, follow the recipes and suggested serving sizes in this book and begin your elimination phase!

3. **You do not have IBS:** As I have mentioned several times throughout this book, you must consult with a doctor, dietician, or nutritionist at least once, if not more regularly, throughout your entire IBS treatment journey. If you have been meeting with a professional, then you will likely have the information you need to try other IBS

treatment options. However, if you haven't seen a professional, and you started the diet on your own and also self-diagnosed yourself with IBS, it is possible that the diet did not work for you because you did not have IBS, to begin with.

Many digestive system disorders can mimic IBS symptoms and make you think your condition is more or less severe than it is. It is possible that you are lactose-intolerant or that you have Celiac disease. It could also mean that you have reproductive system conditions (particularly if you are a woman) or serious IBD that is a potentially fatal autoimmune disease. If you went on the low-FODMAP diet on your own and you were never seen by a doctor, I urge you to make an appointment with a medical professional as soon as you can. This way, you will be able to identify if you have IBS or another condition, and your doctor will place you on the appropriate treatment plan. If it turns out that you do have IBS and trying the low-FODMAP diet did not work for you, please go through the rest of this chapter to see if any of the other scenarios apply to you.

Conclusion

Your gut and I thank you for reaching the end of this book—*The Low-FODMAP Diet*. I hope it was a useful resource for you and was able to provide you with the necessary tools and information you need to achieve your goals.

As a reminder, all of the recipes in this book have been thoroughly reviewed by a variety of dieticians, and each of the recipes is suitable for the elimination phase of the low-FODMAP diet. Many of these recipes are also very customizable, so you can use the same recipes as you transition into phases 2 and 3 after you have finished your elimination phase.

I hope you can share these recipes with friends and family members who may be experiencing IBS gut symptoms, no matter how mild or severe their symptoms may be. All the information in this book is useful to people with varying degrees of IBS, and the low-FODMAP diet is certainly worth your best shot!

My wish is that you can experience a much more comfortable life with the information and recipes from this book and that you can eat to your heart's content without worrying about painful or embarrassing symptoms. Your eating habits should not be compromised because of your IBS symptoms because not eating can be just as bad as eating high-FODMAP foods! I hope you can find a safe ground with these recipes and that you get to experience a whole new world of IBS treatment.

Finally, if you found this book useful in any way, a positive review on Amazon is always appreciated! Thank you, and happy eating!

Book Description:

Welcome to the low-FODMAP diet! This book will be your information guide, encouraging partner, and useful resource as you begin your journey into the low-FODMAP world. Starting this diet can be a little daunting when you first hear about it—you have to eliminate so many day-to-day foods from your diet that it can be hard to know how you will manage to keep yourself fed during this time. Don't fret!

First of all, this book will tell you all about the low-FODMAP diet and how it is NOT a "forever" diet. If you follow the guidelines in the book properly, it is possible that you could be back to eating your favorite high-FODMAP foods in a matter of weeks! This book will teach you about all three phases of the diet, how to follow them properly, and how to begin reintegrating higher-FODMAP ingredients into your diet again. We have provided you with a complete and thoroughly detailed guide of the low-FODMAP diet, so you can be as confident as possible as you begin this treatment for your gut symptoms. In addition to detailing the diet, we have also provided you with information about IBS, its causes, symptoms, and treatments. We hope that you find this extra information beneficial to you in your own IBS journey!

Secondly, this book has a wide variety of recipes that will leave you with many options for meals and snacks that also taste so delicious that you'll forget you're on a diet. We have even listed plenty of options for people who are on vegetarian and vegan diets, so don't feel left out! Each recipe has a description, a list of what you will need, instructions for how to prepare the meal, and a few low-FODMAP shopping tips, so you'll always get the best ingredients for your gut. All the meals in this book will also help you maintain good nutrition while you're on the diet. More tips on how to avoid becoming deficient in particular nutrients are also included in the early chapters of the book. Recipes you can expect to find include:

- Breakfast recipes like smoothies, porridges, and different recipes for eggs. Each of the breakfast recipes will take only 5–10 minutes to make, and some of them can even be prepared the night before. This is for all of you, busy bees!
- Lunch and dinner recipes for our meat lovers include rice, pasta, salads, soups, and other miscellaneous meals. These recipes are filling and have serving sizes that will help you stick to the low-FODMAP guideline. Most of these recipes will yield more than one serving so you can refrigerate and keep the leftovers for later in the week.
- Snack recipes that are more like treats! These goodies will help you between meals, and, believe it or not, they are all low in FODMAP! Some of these snacks are perfect to nibble on throughout the day, but some of them are a little less healthy, so make sure to pay attention to the serving size for each snack!
- Vegetarian and Vegan meals! We have separate sections for vegetarian and vegan recipes because

we recognize that your restrictions are not the same! We also do give some suggestions throughout the main lunch and dinner chapter for making those meals fit your dietary restrictions. You will not be let down by this book if you do not eat meat or other animal products.

We hope you will choose to buy and read this book because we have worked very hard to provide you with the most accurate information and recipes that have been reviewed by personal dieticians. Thank you for checking this out! Good luck with your low-FODMAP journey, and feel free to leave a review, telling us more about how this diet has helped you!

Printed in Great Britain
by Amazon